Yoga Class

8 Essential Yoga Lessons for Beginners

Timothy Burgin

Author of *Yoga For Beginners: A Quick-Start Guide to Practicing Yoga for New Students*

ADHIMUKTI PRESS • 2014

Copyright © 2014 by Timothy Burgin. All rights reserved.

This book or any portion thereof may not be reproduced or used in any manner whatsoever without the express written permission of the publisher except for the use of brief quotations in a book review.

Printed in the United States of America
First Printing, 2014
ISBN 978-0692257197

Editor: Meredith Daniel Sims
Photography, Book Design and Cover Design: Timothy Burgin
Models: Lindsay Fields, Mackenzie Thomas, Annie H. Kim
Clothing: Prana, Wisdomystery

Text set in Baskerville

Adhimukti Press
www.adhimukti.com

Contents

Preface

Before walking into my first yoga class, I was scared and nervous. All I knew about yoga was that you had to be flexible, and I was anything but. Although I was just 19, I could barely touch my knees when bending forward, so the thought of subjecting my body to 90 minutes of various pretzel-like contortions was extremely intimidating. I assumed yoga would be close to impossible for me.

However, my fears and anxieties quickly vanished at the start of my first class. The instructor was warm, friendly and compassionate. She encouraged us to only do what we could, without pushing, pulling, or straining. But most importantly was how she guided our awareness inwards to connect with our breath and the sensations in our bodies as we were practicing the postures.

I found practicing the yoga postures in that first class challenging, but not at all impossible. I quickly learned in my first yoga class that it doesn't matter how far you go into a pose; what matters is doing the pose to your level of ability and with as much awareness of your breathing and body sensations as possible. Not only did I feel a tremendous relief that I could actually do yoga with my inflexible body, but my inflexible body felt amazing after that first class. I was hooked. Over twenty years later, I am still enjoying the physical, mental, and emotional benefits of a regular yoga practice.

I feel so fortunate that I was able to attend class on a regular basis when I started practicing. As the founder and executive director of YogaBasics.com, I hear from many people across the country who want to learn yoga, but who don't have access to a teacher or are too intimidated to join a class. Even those who've tried yoga classes often find that the level of instruction may not be appropriate or adequately address their needs as there are few classes that are geared specifically for beginners. So many beginning students turn to books and websites and start their yoga practice at home.

Although my website, YogaBasics.com, has a lot of content geared specifically towards beginners, I have realized that it might be daunting for new students to try to devise a program on their own. And while there are several good beginner books, this book is the first of its kind that leads the beginning student through a series of lessons to slowly and confidently learn and grow through several weeks of practice.

As a certified Kripalu Yoga teacher, I've been teaching a wide range of students for the last 14 years. I've observed new students from many different populations, from the young college student to the elderly retired person, and have discovered their specific needs and requirements for beginning yoga. All of my experiences with teaching beginning students have helped form the content of this book, as well as my overriding philosophy of keeping instruction simple and basic for beginners.

This book is based on a Yoga for Beginners program that I developed, first as a one-day workshop, and later on as a 6 week series of classes. This not only created the lesson format that forms the core of this book, it also gave me real-world feedback as to how to tailor and refine these lessons to meet the needs of the beginning student. It also gives me the confidence to tell you that this program works. If you diligently practice these lessons over the next several weeks, you will have the skill, strength, ability and confidence to be established in a regular home practice as well as go to a public yoga class.

Introduction

WHAT IS YOGA?

Yoga is a collection of physical and spiritual practices aimed at integrating mind, body, and spirit. The goal of yoga is to achieve a state of inner balance and ultimately, enlightenment (a state of oneness with the universe). There are many different paths of yoga, and what is normally thought of as "yoga" in the West is really hatha yoga, the physical or "forceful" path. In the East, different yogas are practiced that are more focused on devotion, meditation and selfless service. While all of these different paths emphasize different approaches and techniques, they ultimately lead to the same goal of unification and enlightenment.

Though yoga's ultimate aim is lofty, its essence is practical and scientific. Yoga emphasizes direct experience and observable results through a practice of personal inquiry and exploration. While yoga teaches spiritual techniques, it is not religious. As you will discover throughout this book, the philosophy and practice of yoga speaks to universal truths which can be incorporated within any belief system.

HISTORY OF YOGA

The origin of yoga is obscure because of its reliance on oral transmission and secrecy. Early writings were transcribed on fragile palm leaves, which were easily damaged, destroyed, or lost. Most scholars believe yoga originated about 5,000 years ago, but some think that the practice could be up to 10,000 years old.

The practices were developed by the Indus-Sarasvati civilization in Northern India and started in the context of a guru-disciple (teacher-student) relationship. In the ancient days, yogis practiced asceticism and sought to diminish the vitality of the body in order to control desires, which they viewed as an obstacle to liberation. Eventually, some yoga masters began to see the body not as a hindrance to transformation, but as its very vehicle. They created a system of practices designed to balance and energize the body, preparing it for liberation. This philosophy, known as tantra yoga, led to further mind-body explorations, which were the precursor to hatha yoga, the body-centered exercises that are most commonly taught as yoga in the West.

In the 1920s and 30s, hatha yoga was strongly promoted in India through the work of Swami Sivananda, T. Krishnamacharya, and others. Sivananda founded the Divine Life Society on the banks of the holy Ganges River in 1936. A prolific author of over 200 books on yoga, he established nine ashrams and numerous yoga centers worldwide. Krishnamacharya opened the first hatha yoga school in Mysore in 1924. His three most well-known students: B.K.S. Iyengar, T.K.V. Desikachar and Pattabhi Jois, are the founders of Iyengar, Viniyoga, and Ashtanga styles of hatha yoga, all commonly practiced in the West today.

Since then, many more western and Indian teachers have become pioneers, popularizing hatha yoga and gaining millions of followers. Hatha yoga now has many different schools or styles, all emphasizing different aspects of the practice.

HATHA YOGA: THE PHYSICAL PATH

Hatha yoga (ha="sun" tha="moon") attains the union of mind-body-spirit though a practice of asanas (yoga postures), pranayama (yoga breathing), mudra (body gestures) and shatkarma (internal cleansing). These body-centered practices are used to purify the body, cultivate prana, and activate kundalini, the subtle energies of the body. Modern hatha yoga does not emphasize many of these esoteric practices and focuses primarily on the physical yoga postures.

In the history of yoga, hatha yoga is a fairly recent technique that was developed from tantra yoga. The Tantrics embraced the physical body as the means to achieve enlightenment and developed the physical-spiritual connections and body centered practices that lead to hatha yoga. Hatha yoga is uniquely focused on transforming the physical body through purification and the cultivation of the life-force energy of prana. Thus, all of the techniques of hatha yoga are seen as preliminary steps to achieving the deeper states of meditation and enlightenment found in the paths of tantra yoga and raja yoga (meditation).

HOW TO USE THIS BOOK

The core of this book is laid out in a series of eight lessons that slowly and progressively build upon each other. Before the lessons I've included some brief, yet important, introductory information and guidelines on yoga. I have consciously kept the yogic jargon to a minimum and have introduced yogic philosophy only when relevant and needed in the current lesson's practice. While these lessons are intended to be practiced one per week, you can easily move through the book at your own pace. In fact, it would foster your learning and promote a safe learning environment if you did progress at your own time.

In these eight lessons, you will learn 30 of the most commonly used poses that are safe and accessible for the beginning student. You will also learn the basic yoga breathing techniques and simple meditation practices with which to begin and end your yoga sessions. Each lesson will start with the basic practice philosophy and focus on specific principles of alignment. Make sure you understand these guiding concepts as they will be used with the yoga postures to be learned in the practice session of the lesson.

In the eight practice sessions, you will begin the practice of hatha yoga, adding new learned poses with each lesson. We will practice the yoga poses within a sequence that will grow and change as you progress through the lessons. By the end of lesson eight, you will have the skill and confidence to begin modifying and creating your own yoga sequences, or you can continue to follow the sequences that you learned in the practice sessions. In the last chapter of the book, I will give you advice and suggestions on "where to go from here" for those feeling the desire to continue their journey with yoga.

How to Begin Practicing Yoga

GENERAL PRACTICE GUIDELINES

Contraindications: When to Not Practice Yoga

If you have any injuries, recent surgeries, or health conditions, please consult with your physician before beginning a yoga practice. If you have injuries or specific conditions that require modifications, then working with a skilled teacher will be essential to reduce further injury or aggravation of your condition and to promote healing and well-being.

Musculoskeletal Injuries

The basic rule of thumb when working with a joint or muscle injury is to avoid poses that activate pain or aggravate the injury. Once the injury has healed, then one can slowly and cautiously practice poses that work that part of the body again. The following general guidelines do not address musculoskeletal injuries or diseases. For specific assistance with these types of conditions, please consult a qualified yoga teacher or physical therapist.

Pregnancy

During pregnancy it is best not to put any pressure on the abdomen, and to avoid all poses lying on your belly. Modify forward folding poses by having the legs wider apart so the thighs do not press against the abdomen, and modify twists by twisting away from your legs so the legs do not press against the belly. After the first trimester, avoid full inversions, and rest on your side instead of your back during shavasana. (Any posture in which the head is below the heart is called an inversion; a full inversion has the body upside down like headstand or shoulderstand.)

Menstruation

During menstruation it is advised to rest and not to practice yoga or to practice gentle, soothing poses while omitting inversions, backbends, and any strong work with the core muscles of the abdomen and low back.

Modify and Adapt the Postures

It is important to note that the instructions and pictures of the yoga postures are the "goal," meaning the direction you are going towards, not where you need to be. Experiment with and explore different positions and alignment to make the posture work for your body. Use the yoga postures as a mirror to help you see what needs to be changed, modified or adapted for your body. If you need help modifying or adapting the poses to meet the needs of your body, please consult with a qualified yoga instructor.

What to Wear

When selecting clothing to wear during yoga, try to strike a balance between comfort, modesty, and ease of movement. Purchasing specifically designed clothing may be the best route to take if you can afford to do so. If not, you can usually find something in your closet that you already own that will work.

Drinking and Eating

During yoga the abdomen can get compressed and turned upside down. If your stomach is full of food or fluids, it can be very uncomfortable to practice yoga. It is highly recommended that you not eat two hours before your practice and drink minimally before and during your practice.

Duration of Practice

Your daily practice should be between 15 to 90 minutes long and done 1-6 times per week, depending on your schedule, goals and ability. Practicing more frequently with shorter practice times will yield greater results than practicing less frequently with longer practice times. Longer practice times will give you the opportunity to work the entire body as well as go deeper into the experience of yoga.

Intensity of Practice

You can make your yoga practice as challenging and vigorous as you want. I recommend that you start slowly and make sure you understand the alignment of postures. I also highly recommend that you use intensity and challenge as a way to focus the mind and not as a way to strengthen the ego. Ideally you want to have a feeling of radiant health and well-being during your practice and to feel calm and energized after your practice. If you feel tired or exhausted, you are most likely overexerting yourself and need to back off.

Sankalpa - Intention

Creating a sankalpa (intention or prayer) at the beginning of your yoga practice can bring a deeper focus and power, especially if this intention remains active throughout the practice. You can also create individual sankalpas for specific yoga poses to help guide you deeper into these postures. An effective sankalpa is a short, positive, and precise statement about what you wish to attain for yourself and/or for the benefit of all.

"Without intention, all these postures, these breathing practices, meditations, and the like can become little more than ineffectual gestures. When animated by intention, however, the simplest movement, the briefest meditation, and the contents of one breath cycle are made potent."

— Donna Farhi

WHAT YOU WILL NEED TO START

One of the great things about yoga is that you don't really need anything to practice yoga. We do, however, recommend the following to support and enhance your practice:

1. Yoga Mat. A yoga mat provides padding as well as a non-slip surface to practice on. A classic yoga mat is best for beginners, but upgrading to a thicker mat is recommended if you are practicing on a wood floor.

2. Yoga Props. Yoga props are very helpful when starting yoga. Use a yoga block to stabilize standing poses, use a yoga strap to stretch further in seated poses, and use a bolster for restorative poses. Ordinary pillows, blankets, and hardcover books can be used as substitutes for yoga props.

3. Yoga Music. Playing some soft, soothing, and relaxing music while you practice yoga can block out distractions and help you focus and be more present.

Exploring the Spine and Breath

THE YOGIC BREATH

I always tell new students that the most important thing to do in yoga is to breathe. The breath is the canary in the coal mine: if you cannot maintain a slow deep breath during yoga then something is wrong! If you find yourself holding your breath or not able to take a slow deep breath, then you need to back out of the pose, modify the pose, or come out completely.

The breath is considered the foundation of the practice of yoga, and using slow deep yogic breathing is one of the major differences between yoga and other forms of exercise. The importance of maintaining this yogic breath is emphasized by the yogic teaching that says we are each born with only a certain number of breaths. Therefore, to extend the length of our lives we just need to slow down our breathing.

Granted, that can seem a bit simplistic and naive, but modern science shows that there is some truth to that ancient theory. Breathing slowly and deeply activates the parasympathetic nervous system, or the rest and renew response, which reduces stress and allows the body to heal. (The opposite of the rest and renew response is the fight or flight stress response of the sympathetic nervous system.) Because medical research has shown that stress is the number one contributing factor in most diseases, it would not be difficult to believe that minimizing stress through slow deep breathing could indeed help prolong your life.

PRANAYAMA

The ancient yogis explored and developed many different breathing practices that they called pranayama. Prana is a Sanskrit word that translates into "life force energy" and yama can be translated as the "control or mastery of." Thus, pranayama is used to control, cultivate, and modify the life force energy that is present in the air we breathe. While it is a separate practice, pranayama can also be combined with asana, the practice of yoga postures. In this book, we will learn two pranayamas commonly used with asana to increase stamina, concentration, and energy.

Dirga Pranayama - The Three Part Breath

The first pranayama we will learn is called Dirga Pranayama. Known as the "three part" or "complete" breath, it is the foundation of all of the breathing practices done in yoga. Dirga Pranayama is called the three part breath because you are actively breathing into three parts of your torso. This full, deep breath uses the diaphragm as the primary muscle of respiration and is the most efficient way to breathe. The diaphragm drops down into the lower abdomen on the inhalation, pressing the belly outwards and contracts upwards towards the chest on the exhalation. This movement massages the internal organs and activates the relaxation response in the body.

As with many practices in yoga, what may sound or look easy can be quite challenging and difficult, and mastering the three part breath is no exception. For many students, it can take up to a year to "get it" because most of us have adopted patterns of constricted or reverse pattern breathing. Struggling to maintain a full, deep breath throughout the practice is normal for beginning students. So be steadfast in your resolve to master Dirga, but also be compassionate with yourself, acknowledging the time and effort needed to feel comfortable with breathing in this new way.

We will explore this breath in further detail in this lesson's practice session.

THE SPINE

Yoga is a unique form of physical exercise by its emphasis on the health, strength, and flexibility of the spine. This is summarized by the yoga proverb: "You are as only as young as your spine is flexible."

The spine (vertebral column or backbone) is an interconnected column of 24 vertebrae, separated by spongy disks, and are categorized into four sections:

Cervical - seven vertebrae of the neck

Thoracic - twelve vertebrae supporting the ribcage

Lumbar - five vertebrae of the low back

Sacrum – five bones fused together to form a single boney plate

There are three natural curves of the spine: cervical, thoracic and lumbar. Looking at the spine from the side, these three curves resemble a gentle "S" shape. These curves function to distribute the mechanical stress created when the body is both moving and at rest. Abnormal or excessive curving of the spine results in pain, limited functionality, and poor posture. Yoga naturally maintains and strengthens the three natural curves in the body through the six movements of the spine.

The Six Movements of the Spine

The spine can move in six directions: arching (extension) and rounding (flexion), twisting left and right (rotation), and side-bending to the left and right (lateral flexion). Most yoga poses activate one of these movements, and some postures move the spine in more than one direction. Each of these six movements has a different effect on the spine as well as the muscles surrounding it.

A yoga practice should contain all six movements of the spine to create a sense of balance and completeness. Each practice session does not need to have an equal amount of these movements, but should include at least one pose that moves the spine in each of these directions. These six movements take the spine through its entire range of motion, as well as help to naturally re-align the vertebrae and maintain the proper alignment of the spine. Without moving through all six movements there will be a feeling of incompleteness, and you will not receive the full benefits of yoga's effect on the spine.

The Breath and the Spine

There is actually a seventh movement of the spine: a subtle lengthening of the entire vertebral column called axial extension. In yoga, the six movements of the spine are usually practiced with axial extension as this lengthening creates the greatest range of movement in the spine.

This lengthening action is often linked with the breath. The proper full yogic breath expands the torso in three dimensions and naturally lengthens the spine with an inhalation. So when moving into the yoga poses, it feels natural to lengthen the spine on the inhalation and then to move the spine in one of the six directions on the exhalation. It also feels natural to inhale while arching the spine (extension) and to exhale while rounding the spine (flexion).

PRACTICE SESSION

In this lesson's practice we will start with Easy Pose and use this basic seated position to learn and practice Dirga Pranayama. After practicing the warm-up sequence one or more times, we'll end with the relaxing Shavasana pose.

Easy Pose or Sukhasana

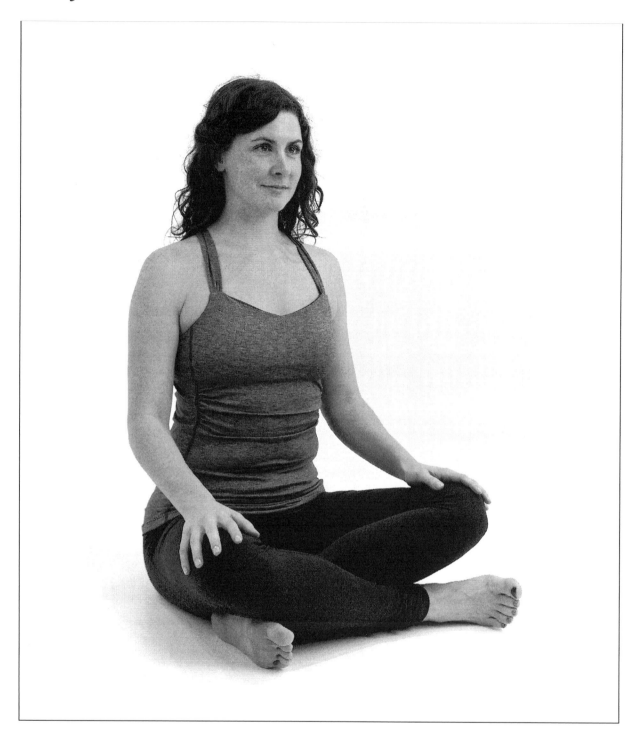

I like to come into Easy Pose at the beginning and end of every yoga practice. This is an easeful, seated pose to prepare for yoga practice by drawing the focus inwards. Taking a few breaths in Easy Pose at the end of a practice is a gentle way to transition from your yoga practice to being back in the world.

Instructions

1. Come into a seated position with the buttocks on the floor, then cross the legs, placing the feet directly below the knees. Rest the hands on the knees or the lap with the palms facing up or down.

2. Press the sitting bones down into the floor, and reach the crown of the head up to lengthen the spine. Drop the shoulders down and back, and press the chest towards the front of the room.

3. Relax the face, jaw, and belly. Let the tongue rest on the roof of the mouth, just behind the front teeth.

4. Breathe deeply through the nose and down into the belly. Hold for a few minutes or as long as comfortable.

Benefits: Easy pose is a comfortable seated position for meditation. This pose opens the hips, lengthens the spine, and promotes groundedness and inner calm.

Contraindications: Recent or chronic knee or hip injury or inflammation.

Modifications: Place folded blanket under knees or under the sitting bones.

Note: Begin every yoga practice session with this pose.

Practicing Dirga Pranayama

To practice Dirga Pranayama, we will be actively breathing into three parts of your abdomen. The first position is the low belly (on top of or just below the belly button), the second position is the low chest (lower half of the rib cage), and the third position is the upper chest (just below the collar bones). The breath is continuous, inhaled and exhaled through the nose. The inhalation starts in the first position (the low belly), then moves to the second position (the low chest). then to the third position (the upper chest). The exhalation starts in the upper chest, moves to the low chest, and finishes in the low belly.

To practice, stay in Easy Pose or Sukhasana (the pose we just learned) with one had on the low belly and the other hand on the low chest. Inhale into the low belly, and feel the breath rising against your hand. Exhale, and feel the hand sinking back in towards the belly. Once you have a good feel for this, then work on feeling the inhale and exhale in the first and second positions. Once you can feel the breath in the first and second positions, move the upper hand to the upper chest and work on feeling the inhale and exhale in all three positions. Lastly, allow the hands to rest on your knees or lap and continue to feel the breath moving in all three positions. Eventually relax the effort of the Pranayama, and breathe into the three positions gently, feeling a wave of breath move up and down the torso.

Warm-Up Sequence

In this lesson this warm-up sequence will be practiced by itself, but in future lessons it is best used after the starting meditation and before practicing the yoga poses. Use gentle, fluid movements synchronized with slow, deep breathing to prepare the muscles and joints for moving into and holding the yoga poses. For a deeper effect, you can hold each stretch for 1-2 breaths or repeat these warm-ups multiple times. This sequence is contraindicated with recent or chronic injury to the arms, neck or back.

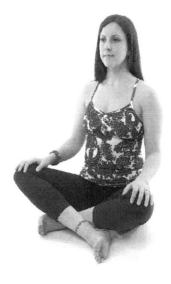

1. Start in Easy Pose.

Keep the shoulders down and back, the spine long, and the chest open.

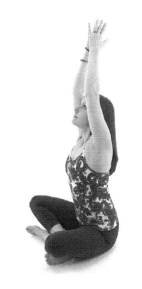

2. Inhale the fingertips up to the ceiling.

Keep the shoulders down and back, the hips grounded to the floor, and reach through the fingertips.

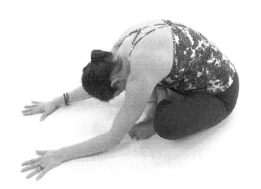

3. Exhale and round forward with the palms to the floor.

Round the spine, and relax the head and elbows down.

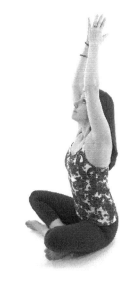

4. Inhale the fingertips up to the ceiling.

Keep the shoulders down and back, the hips grounded to the floor, and reach through the fingertips.

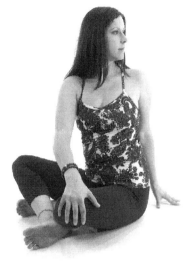

5. Exhale and twist to the left.

Place the left hand on the right knee and the right hand behind your back. Look over your right shoulder, and look behind you. Keep the spine long and the shoulders down.

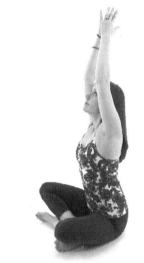

6. Inhale the fingertips up to the ceiling.

Keep the shoulders down and back, the hips grounded to the floor, and reach through the fingertips.

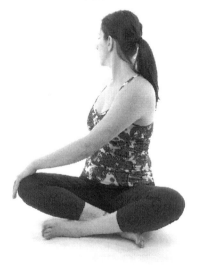

7. Exhale and twist to the right.

Place the right hand on the left knee and the left hand behind your back. Look over your left shoulder, and look behind you. Keep the spine long and the shoulders down.

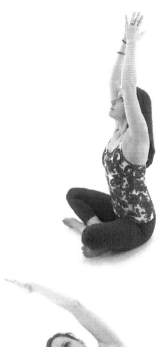

8. Inhale the fingertips up to the ceiling.

Keep the shoulders down and back, the hips grounded to the floor, and reach through the fingertips.

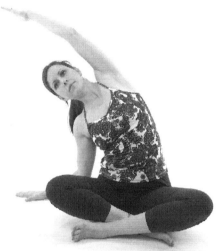

9. Exhale the left hand to the floor, and arch to the left.

Reach out through the right fingers, and lower the left elbow as close to the floor as comfortable. Keep the chin off the chest and the right arm over the right ear.

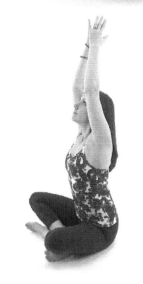

10. Inhale the fingertips up to the ceiling.

Keep the shoulders down and back, the hips grounded to the floor, and reach through the fingertips.

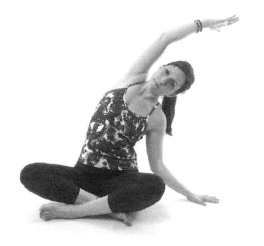

11. Exhale the right hand to the floor and arch to the right.

Reach out through the left fingers, and lower the right elbow as close to the floor as comfortable. Keep the chin off the chest and the right arm over the left ear.

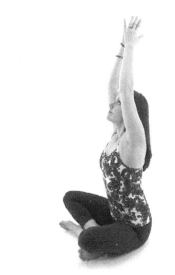

12. Inhale the fingertips up to the ceiling.

Keep the shoulders down and back, the hips grounded to the floor, and reach through the fingertips.

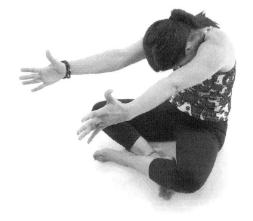

13. Exhale the hands forward, and round the spine.

Reach out through the fingertips, drop the head down, and round the spine.

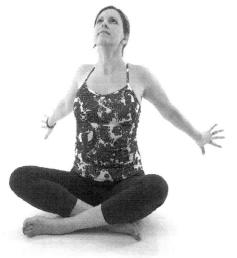

14. Inhale the arms behind you.

Reach back through the fingertips to draw the shoulder blades together. Press forward through the chest, and look up towards the ceiling.

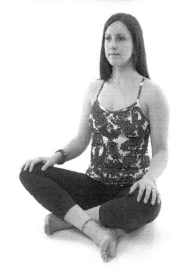

15. Exhale the hands to the knees or floor.

Bring the spine back to neutral position. Keep the shoulders down and back, the spine long, and the chest open.

Corpse or Shavasana

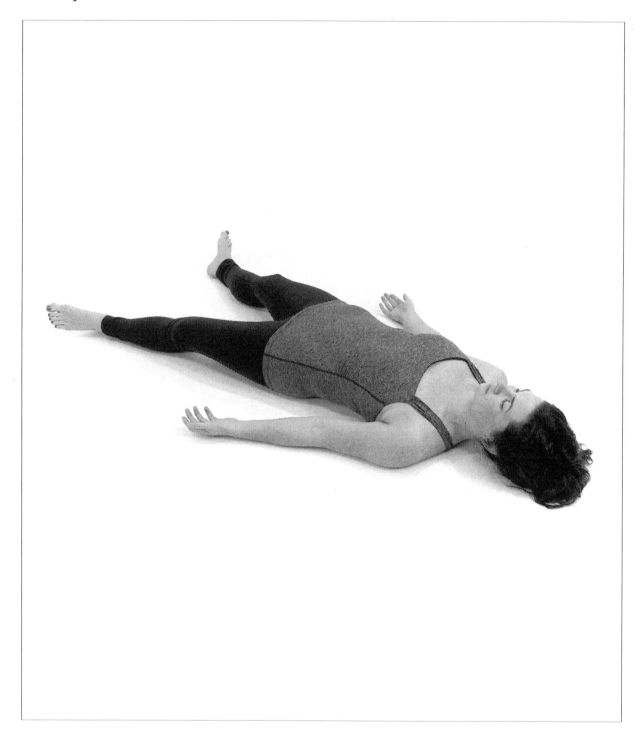

In this pose we "play dead," letting the body lie still and be completely relaxed. At first, spending a few minutes in this pose will feel like an eternity, but once you learn how delicious it is to completely let go and be present with the body and breath you will savor these last minutes of your practice.

Instructions

1. Lying on your back, let the arms and legs drop open with the arms about 45 degrees from the side of your body. Make sure you are warm and comfortable. If you need to, place blankets under or over your body.

2. Close the eyes, and take slow deep breaths through the nose. Allow your whole body to become soft and heavy, relaxing into the floor. As the whole body relaxes, feel it rising and falling with each breath.

3. Scan the body from the toes to the fingers to the crown of the head, looking for tension, tightness and contracted muscles. Consciously release and relax any areas that you find. If you need to, rock or wiggle part of your body from side to side to encourage further release.

4. Release all control of the breath, the mind, and the body. Let your body move deeper and deeper into a state of total relaxation.

5. Stay in Shavasana for 5 to 15 minutes.

6. To release, slowly deepen the breath, wiggle the fingers and toes, reach the arms over your head and stretch the whole body. Exhale, bend the knees into the chest, and roll over to one side coming into a fetal position. When you are ready, slowly inhale up to a seated position.

Benefits: Corpse pose is essential to practice at the end of every yoga practice. This posture rejuvenates the body, mind and spirit while reducing stress and tension.

Contraindications: Third trimester of pregnancy.

Modifications: Place a bolster or blankets under the low back and/or knees.

Note: End every yoga practice session with this pose.

LESSON TWO

Creating the Foundation

AHIMSA, NON-HARMING OR NON-VIOLENCE

Ahimsa is the practice of non-harming, which includes physical, mental, and emotional violence towards others and oneself. Taken in this broad context, ahimsa can feel like an overwhelming practice to take on, but as with any yoga practice, it is best to start simply and slowly. And the best place to start is on our yoga mats! We can apply the concept of ahimsa to how compassionately we treat our bodies, the level of engagement we choose to use in yoga poses, and how well we "stay on the edge" in the poses.

Go to Your Edge

When holding a yoga posture, go right to your edge, but no further. The edge is the place where you feel a deep stretch and/or you feel that the body is working hard, but there is no pain or strain. This edge may be intense, but do not push past it into discomfort or pain; this is where you could hurt yourself or cause undue stress to the body. Once you find the edge in a yoga pose, stay there and consciously breathe deeply. With every inhalation, recharge the pose by activating the muscles to refine to your alignment, and with every exhalation, relax into the pose by consciously releasing the muscles you are not using. You may find that if you can relax into the edge, it will slowly back away, at which point you can follow it to move deeper into the pose.

KARUNA, THE PRACTICE OF COMPASSION

Compassion is an aspect of ahimsa that can be practiced mentally, emotionally and physically in your yoga practice. Our minds often respond to being challenged in a yoga pose with negative thoughts of judging, complaining, criticizing, and comparing. This response is so ingrained in us that we may not even be aware of our harmful chatter of "I can't do this" or "I'm so inflexible" or "I suck at this pose." To counteract this, work on cultivating mindful awareness and an attitude of optimism and self-compassion in your yoga practice.

When you come into a pose, notice what the mind is saying, and try to catch it during or just before any harmful thoughts arise. Let go of any harmful thoughts as quickly as possible, directing the focus of your mind back to the breath and the physical sensations in the body. Work towards creating a circle of acceptance and compassion around yourself with each breath that you take.

I often tell my students: "Yoga is a journey – this practice is a constantly evolving and ongoing process. Yoga is not about attaining the perfect pose, it's about feeling the aliveness, mystery, and excitement in this moment." For the most part, everyone feels about the same stretch and sensations when practicing a yoga pose, and everyone is receiving the same benefit no matter where they are in the pose, as long as they are at their "edge." The inner aspect of a pose--how much presence and awareness someone is bringing to their practice--is the most important aspect of yoga. The journey of yoga is to be as completely present, accepting, and compassionate as possible to what your body can do in each moment.

THE SPINE AND THE PELVIS

The pelvis is a bowl-shaped structure of three different bones that support the spinal column and connect it to the legs. The pelvis is commonly referred to as the hips, and the hip joint is the connection of the leg bones to the pelvis. Because the sacrum is both considered part of the spine and part of the pelvis, any movement of the pelvis will directly effect the movement of the spine, and vice versa.

There are four movements of the pelvis that effect the movement of the spine: tilting the pelvis from side to side (lateral flexion) and tilting the pelvis forward (anteversion) and backward (retroversion). In this practice session, we will focus on the forward and backward tilting of the pelvis and how this helps to arch and round the spine.

PRACTICE SESSION: A FOUNDATIONAL SEQUENCE

Traditionally, a hatha yoga practice is composed of a sequence of poses. While the possible combinations of poses is limitless, there is an intelligent and orderly way to sequence a yoga session. In this lesson's practice session, we will explore a foundational sequence of 10 poses that will form the basic outline from which we will build upon and add to throughout this book.

Start your practice with the warm-up sequence we learned in the first lesson, and practice Dirga Pranayama at the beginning and/or end of this lesson's session. You can repeat low warrior immediately after the first side or you can go back through the sequence to repeat low warrior with the opposite leg.

FOUNDATIONAL SEQUENCE OVERVIEW

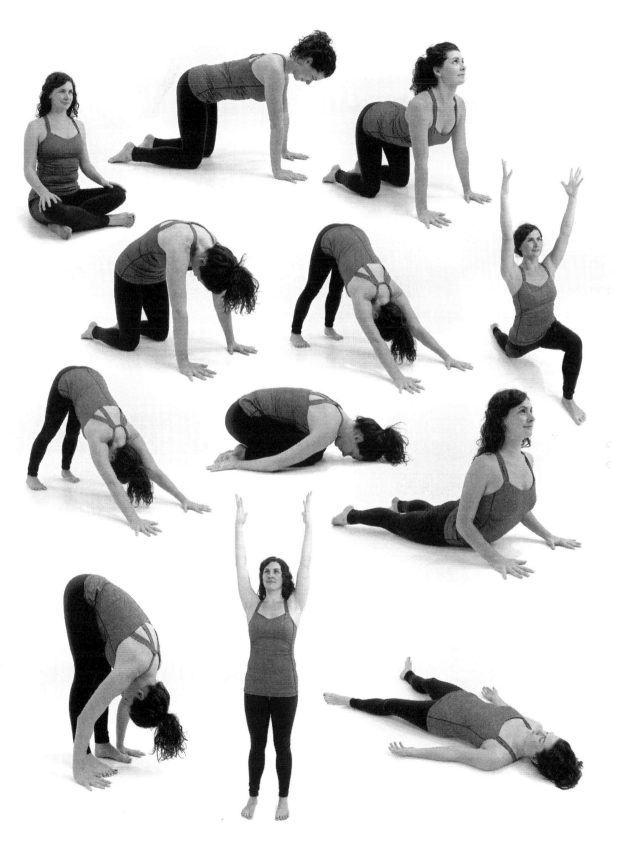

Table Pose or Bharmanasana

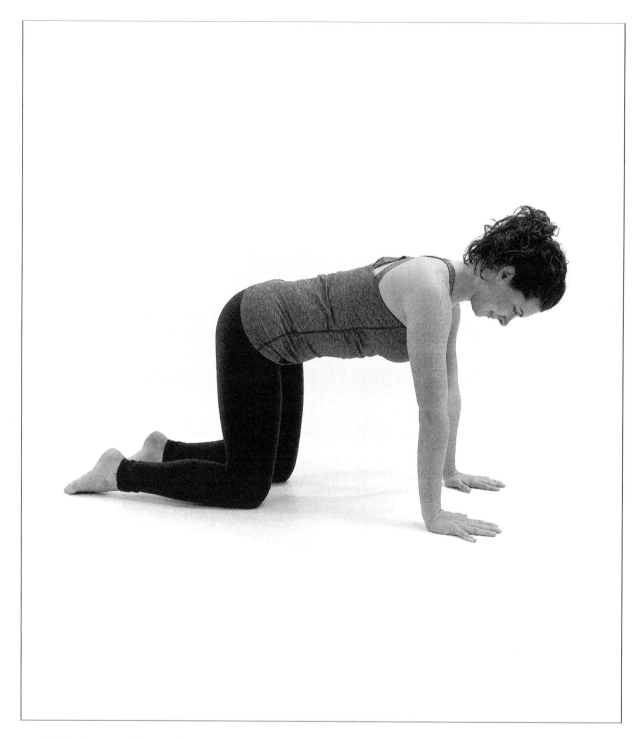

Table is a good transition pose, but holding the pose for a few breaths can lengthen and help realign the spine. The alignment principles in the hands, shoulders and spine will be applicable to downward facing dog.

Instructions

1. Come to the floor on your hands and knees. Bring the knees hip width apart, with the feet directly behind the knees. Bring the palms directly under the shoulders with the fingers facing forward.

2. Look down between the palms and allow the back to be flat. Press out into the fingertips to decrease the weight in the wrists. Slide the shoulders towards the waist, reach the sternum forward and gently pull the navel up. Reach the tail bone towards the back wall and the crown of the head towards the front wall to lengthen the spine.

3. Breathe deeply and hold for 2-3 breaths.

Benefits: Table is the starting point and transition posture for many floor postures and helps lengthen and realign the spine.

Contraindications: Recent or chronic injury to the wrists or knees.

Modifications: A) Place a folded blanket under the knees to protect them from pressure and stress. B) Make fists with the hands to reduce pressure on the wrists.

Dog Tilt Pose or Svanasana

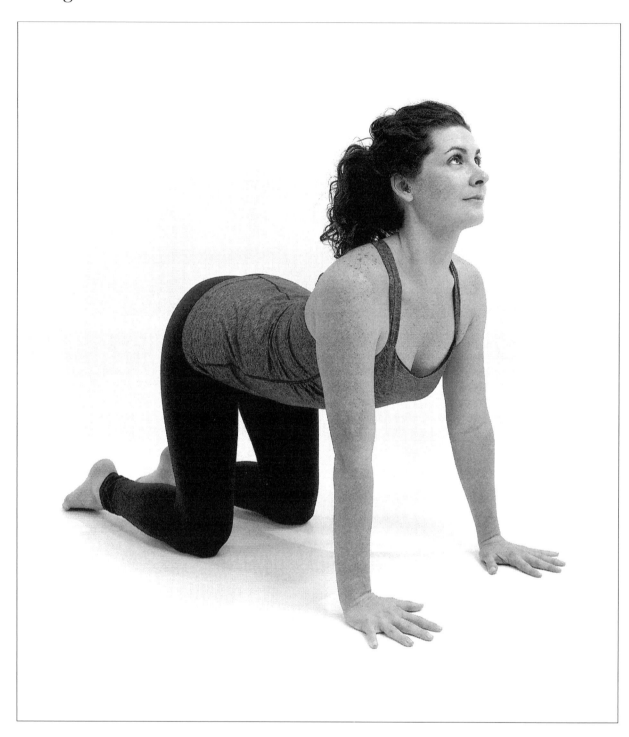

Dog tilt is a gentle back bending pose and, in combination with cat tilt pose, helps to warm up and stretch the back muscles.

Instructions

1. From table pose, inhale and reach the tailbone up towards the ceiling, arching the spine and letting the belly drop down.

2. Spread the fingers wide apart, and press out into the fingertips to decrease the weight in the wrists. Slide the shoulders towards your waist, and reach the crown of the head up towards the ceiling. Look up as high as you can towards the ceiling without straining the back of the neck.

3. Breathe and hold for 4-8 breaths, or move with the breath, inhaling into dog and exhaling into our next asana, cat tilt pose.

4. To release, exhale and flatten the back, moving into table or child pose.

Benefits: Dog tilt pose stretches the middle to low back and hips, lengthens the spine, and stimulates the kidneys and adrenal glands.

Contraindications: Recent or chronic back pain or injury.

Modifications: Place a folded blanket under the knees to protect them.

Cat Tilt Pose or Marjariasana

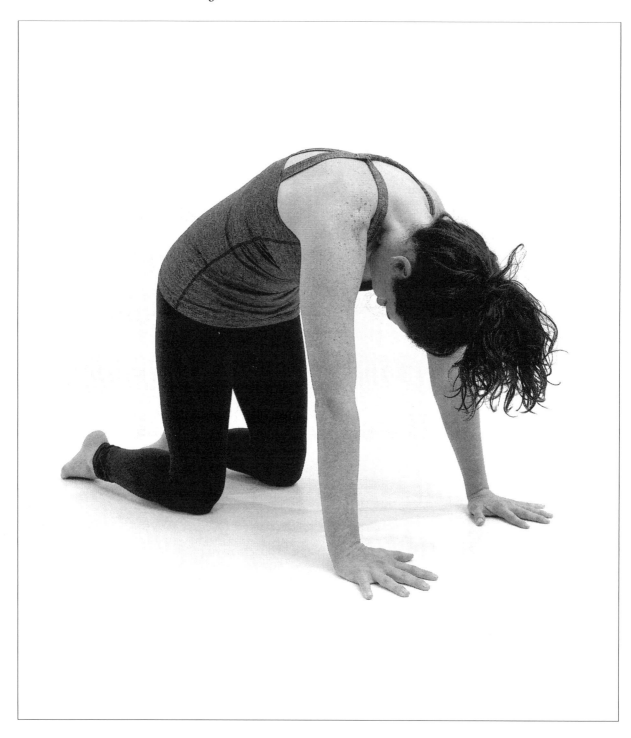

Cat tilt is the complementary pose to dog tilt. Pay attention to the tucking under action of the tailbone here as this is a common, yet often confusing, alignment cue in yoga.

Instructions

1. From table pose, exhale and tuck the tail bone under. Round the spine, and let the head relax down towards the floor.

2. Press out into the fingertips to decrease the weight in the wrists, and reach the middle and upper back up towards the ceiling.

3. Breathe and hold for 4-8 breaths, or vinyasa between cat pose and dog pose, inhaling into dog and exhaling into cat.

4. To release, inhale and flatten the back, moving into table.

Benefits: Cat pose stretches the middle to upper back and shoulders.

Contraindications: Recent or chronic back pain or injury.

Modifications: Place a folded blanket under the knees to protect them.

Downward Facing Dog or Adho Mukha Shvanasana

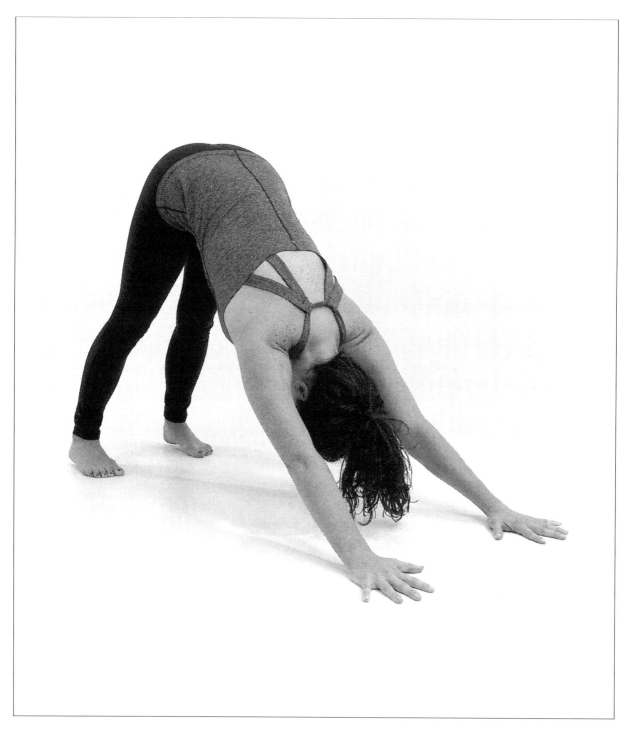

Downward facing dog is the primary transition pose to move from seated to standing poses. I love to do this pose at the end of a long day in front of the computer as it realigns my spine, opens up my shoulders, and stretches the back side of my body.

Instructions

1. From table position, walk the hands six inches forward, tuck the toes under, press into the hands and begin to lift the hips up towards the ceiling.

2. Spread the fingers wide apart with the middle finger facing forward and the palms shoulder width apart. Press out through the fingers and edges of the hands to minimize the weight in the wrists.

3. Using straight (but not locked) arms, press the hips up and back reaching the chest towards the thighs. Lift up through the tailbone to keep the spine straight and long.

4. Have the feet hip width apart with the toes facing forward. Press the heels towards the floor, feeling a stretch in the back of the legs. The legs are straight, or you can have a small bend at the knees to keep the back flat.

5. Let the head and neck hang freely from the shoulders, or align the ears with the arms and reach the crown of the head towards the thumbs.

6. Breathe and hold for 4-8 breaths.

7. To release, bend the knees and lower the hips back to table position, or come all the way down to child pose.

Benefits: Downward facing dog deeply stretches the back and leg muscles, and builds upper body strength. This posture stimulates the brain and nervous system, improving memory, concentration, hearing and eyesight.

Contraindications: Recent or chronic injury to the back, hips, arms or shoulders, or unmedicated high blood pressure.

Modifications: A) Use blocks under the hands or head. B) Place a folded towel under the wrists. C) Press both heels against a wall.

Low Warrior I or Ardha Virabhadrasana I

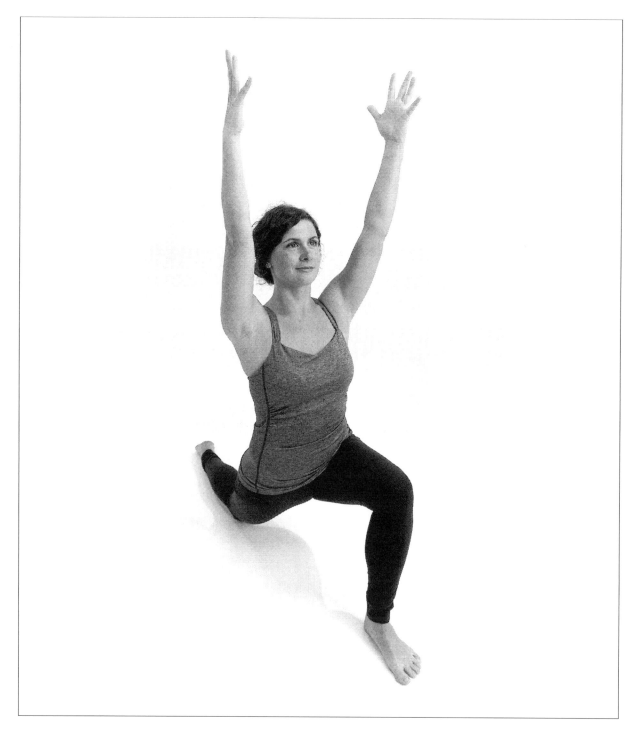

In this pose, we work to find a balance between grounding down through a strong foundation and reaching up with open shoulders and length in the arms and spine. See if you can invoke a powerful and courageous warrior energy in this pose.

Instructions

1. From table pose or downward facing dog pose, step the right foot forward between the two hands, with the knee directly over the ankle.

2. With the legs grounding into the floor, place the hands on the front knee. Straighten the arms slightly to draw the torso back. Relax the shoulders down, and draw the shoulder blades towards the spine to lift the chest.

3. Inhale the arms slowly up over the head in an "H" position or with the palms facing. If you wish to take the pose deeper, bring the palms together, look up and arch back. Keep the arms aligned next to the ears to keep the back of the neck long.

4. Breathe and hold for 2-6 breaths.

5. To release, exhale and bring the palms back to the floor on opposite sides of the right foot, and step the right foot back into table pose or downward facing dog.

6. Repeat on the other side.

Benefits: This pose tones the lower body, and opens the shoulders and hips. Low Warrior I pose also improves focus, balance and concentration.

Contraindications: Recent or chronic injury to the arms, hips, ankles or shoulders.

Modifications: A) Place a folded blanket under the knees. B) Keep the hands on the bent knee.

Child Pose or Balasana

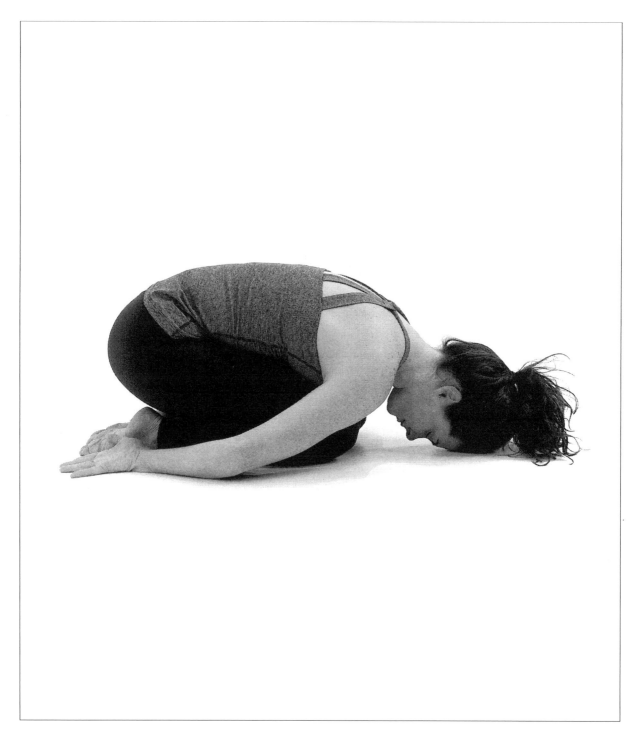

Come into child pose whenever you need to rest or to rejuvenate after a backbend or strenuous pose. This pose creates an opportunity to reflect on your practice and integrate effects of the postures.

Instructions

1. From table or downward facing dog, exhale and lower the hips to the heels and forehead to the floor. Have the knees together or if more comfortable, spread the knees slightly apart.

2. The arms can be overhead with the palms on the floor, the palms or fists can be stacked under the forehead, or the arms can be alongside the body with the palms facing up.

3. Breathe slowly and deeply, actively pressing the belly against the thighs on the inhale. If the low back feels tense you can slowly rock the hips from side to side.

4. Breathe and hold for 4-12 breaths.

5. To release, place the palms under the shoulders and slowly inhale up to a seated position.

Benefits: Child pose calms the body, mind and spirit and stimulates the third eye point. Child pose gently stretches the low back, massages and tones the abdominal organs, and stimulates digestion and elimination.

Contraindications: Recent or chronic injury to the knees.

Modifications: A) Place a blanket under the hips, knees and/or head. B) If pregnant, spread the knees wide apart to remove any pressure on the abdomen.

Variations: Open the knees wider to slide the arms between the legs reaching under the body and turn the head to the side.

Other Names: This pose is also known as embryo/garbhasana/or hare/ Shashankasana.

Cobra or Bhujangasana

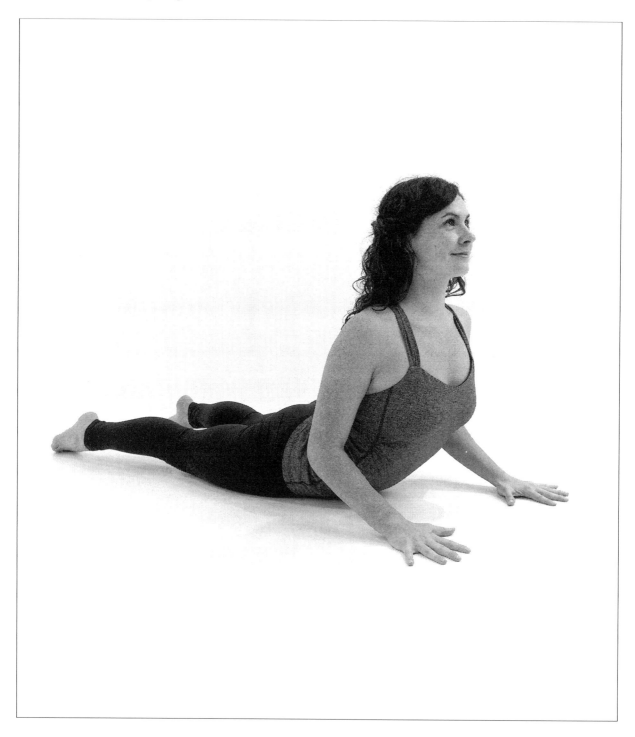

This is the most practiced back-bending pose in yoga. See if you can let this pose feel invigorating and exciting rather than a challenge or struggle. Try lifting the corners of the mouth to bring a bit of light-heartedness and joy into this strenuous pose.

Instructions

1. Lie on your belly with the chin on the floor, palms flat on the floor under the shoulders, and legs together.

2. Press the pubic bone and the tops of the feet down into the floor. Without using the arms, inhale and lift the head and chest off of the floor, keeping the neck in line with the spine.

3. With the elbows close to your sides, press down into the palms and use the arms to lift you up even higher. Drop the shoulders down and back, and press the chest forward. Keep the legs, and buttocks strong, and keep the pubic bone and the tops of the feet pressing down into the floor.

4. Draw the chin in towards the center of the neck, and look up to the forehead with the back of the neck long. Press out through the fingertips and reach out through the toes.

5. Breathe and hold for 2-6 breaths.

6. To release, exhale and slowly lower the chest and head to the floor. Turn the head to one side and rest. Rock the hips from side to side to release any tension in the low back.

Benefits: Cobra opens the chest and strengthens the core body. Cobra aligns the spine and invigorates the kidneys and nervous system.

Contraindications: Recent or chronic injury to the back, arms or shoulders, pregnancy or recent abdominal surgery.

Modifications: To reduce strain in the low back and make the pose less intense: A) Increase the bend in the elbows, or B) Walk the hands further forward.

Standing Forward Fold or Uttanasana

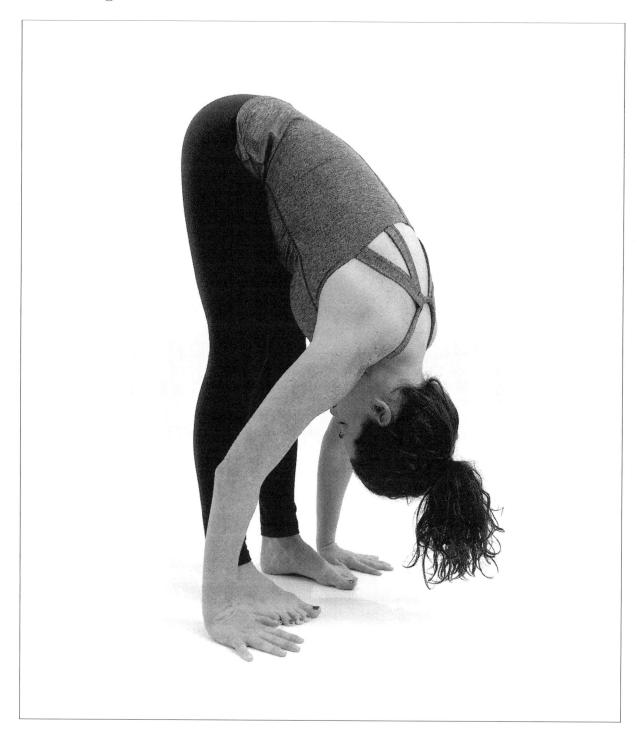

Standing forward fold is a transitional pose that invites you to look deeply within. This is one of the best poses to practice the yogic principle of ahimsa (non-harming). Resist the temptation to push and pull yourself into the pose; instead work on relaxing into the aliveness of the stretch.

Instructions

1. From mountain pose, exhale, hinging forward at the hips, and let the arms sweep out to the sides. Bend the knees enough to bring the fingertips or the palms to the floor, and press the head towards the knees. (If you have low back issues, keep the back perfectly flat in this pose.)

2. Feel the spine stretching in opposite directions as you gently reach the head down and in, and press the hips up. Work on straightening the legs to deepen the stretch in the backs of the legs.

3. Breathe and hold for 4-8 breaths, actively pressing the belly into the thighs on the inhalation.

4. To release, bend the knees, keeping the back straight. Inhale the arms out to the sides, and inhale the arms and torso back up into mountain pose.

Benefits: Standing forward fold pose lengthens the spinal column and deeply stretches the backs of the legs and the back muscles.

Contraindications: Recent or chronic injury to the legs, hips, back or shoulders.

Modifications: Place yoga blocks under the hands.

Variations: There are multiple variations on the placement of the hands: A) Hold on to the backs of the ankles, B) Scoop the fingers under the feet until the toes reach the wrists, C) Cross the arms behind the legs and hold onto the front of the ankles with opposite hands, D) Clasp the elbows behind the legs.

Mountain or Tadasana

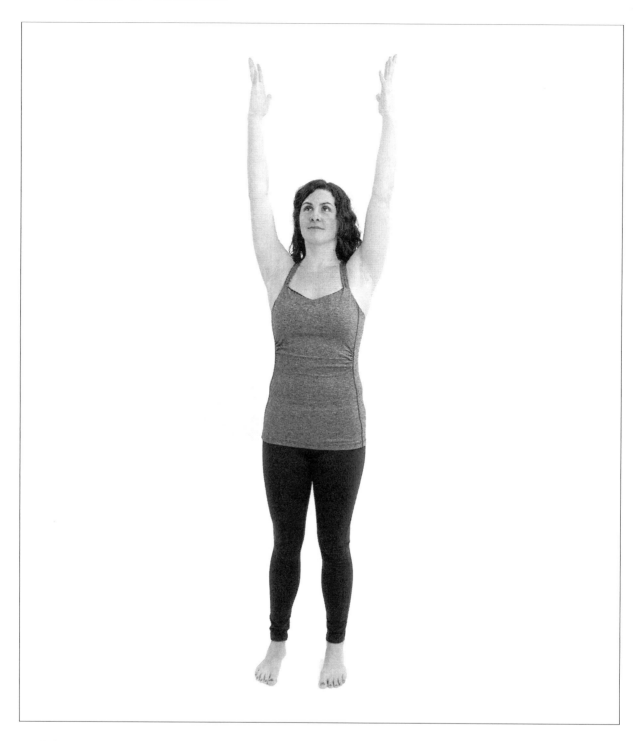

Mountain is the foundation for all of the standing poses in yoga. This pose also encourages us to feel a strong connection to the earth below as well as to the energy of the heavens above. While this may look like an easy pose, I'd encourage you to take the time to master the alignment principles in Mountain pose to fully benefit from its effects.

Instructions

1. From a standing position, bring the feet about hip width apart and parallel. Spread the toes apart, and line up the hips, shoulders and head over the ankles so the weight presses evenly through the bottoms of the feet.

2. Very lightly press the toes down, just enough to feel the muscles of the feet engage. Then pull up the knee caps, squeeze the thighs, and hug the tailbone and navel slightly towards each other.

3. Inhale and lift out of the waist, and reach the crown of the head up towards the ceiling with a long and straight spine.

4. Exhale and release the shoulders down and back, and turn the palms slightly forward. Inhale and reach the fingertips towards the floor, and gently reach the chest/sternum forward slightly. Hold here for a breath or two.

5. Continuing to reach out through the fingers, slowly inhale the arms up into an "H" position.

6. Exhale and relax the shoulders down from the ears while still reaching the crown and fingers up. If you need to further relax the shoulders, you can have the arms in a "Y" shape.

7. Breathe and hold for 3-6 breaths.

8. To release, exhale the arms down to your sides, or bring the palms together in front of your chest.

Benefits: Mountain pose is the foundation for all the standing postures, and it improves posture, groundedness, stability, and confidence.

Contraindications: Recent or chronic injury to the shoulders.

Variations: There are multiple variations on the placement of the hands: A) Fingers interlaced with index finger pointing up, B) Arms down with the palms resting against the outer thighs, C) Palms together in front of the heart in anjali mudra (prayer position).

Standing Strong

ABHYASA: RIGHT EFFORT, WILLFUL ACTION

Abhyasa, right effort and willful action, is an essential element needed to hold strengthening poses with proper alignment for more than a few breaths. The introduction of standing poses in this chapter will require an active engagement of our muscles to produce the "right effort" in the pose: just enough contraction to attain a willful alignment, but not over-engaging the muscles to produce tension and tightness in the body.

When we actively hold a pose, we create a controlled stressful event in the body, and this naturally prompts the body to respond in habitual patterns to stress: tensing the face and jaw, hunching the shoulders, shortening the breath, etc. When sustaining a standing posture, we must be mindful of the effort and engagement of the muscles and adjust the effort to match only what is required by the pose, relaxing any muscles that are not needed. By consciously holding the poses using a balanced amount of engagement and with a slow, deep breath we begin to re-train our natural response to stress. This training of right effort and willful action will make the yoga poses more effective and enjoyable as well as reducing stress both on and off the mat. Since habitual patterns to stress are deeply ingrained, it takes a regular and constant yoga practice, a conscious and consistent inquiry of abhyasa in each pose, to slowly reprogram these patterns.

Create a Strong Foundation

Like a house, a strong and stable standing yoga pose must be built from the foundation up. To create this, we must stack the bones under one another by properly aligning the major joints of the body. Always start your standing poses by rooting the feet into the floor and then aligning the knees properly over the ankles. Build on the base of the feet by engaging the muscles of the legs to support the alignment of the pelvis directly over the feet and to further ground the lower body into the earth. Once the foundation of the lower body is established, then we can confidently build our standing poses by lengthening the spine and reaching through the fingers to lengthen the arms. When the foundation is created properly, the lower body feels solid and stable, and the upper body will have a feeling of lightness and openness.

THE FEET AND THE KNEES

To properly engage the foundation in the standing poses, we must learn to root the feet into the earth. To do this, find the three anchor points of the feet: the heel, the ball of the big toe and the base of the pinky toe. (These three points are the connection points for the three arches of the feet.) Press the anchor points down evenly into the floor, finding a perfect balance in each foot. You may want to move the hips and upper body forward, back and side-to-side to feel the weight shifting and to slowly find the balance between the points. Also, work on balancing the weight of the body evenly between the two feet. The inner arches of the feet should then be lifted away from the floor by spreading these three points away from each other and by lifting the kneecaps and engaging the muscles of the inner legs.

The knees are delicate joints, and awareness must be given to them in poses that focus on the legs, especially the standing poses. The knee is a hinge joint, but when it is bent it becomes destabilized and can twist slightly from side to side. This twisting action can torque the knee and strain the joint and its tendons and ligaments, especially when stress is added to the twisting movement. Because of this, the knee should always track directly forward towards the middle toe and never twist from side to side.

The knee can also be strained in other positions. In lunging poses the knee should be directly over the ankle, not going over the toes. In standing poses with the legs straight, keep the knees just slightly bent to avoid locking and hyperextending the knees.

PRACTICE SESSION: STANDING SEQUENCE

In this practice session we focus on the common standing poses used in yoga. Start your practice with the warm-up sequence we learned in the first lesson, and practice Dirga Pranayama at the beginning and/or end of this lesson's session.

After the warm-up sequence we will start in mountain pose, as its alignment is applicable to many of the poses you are about to learn. For the warrior I, warrior II and triangle poses you can either repeat them on the other side immediately after the first, or repeat the sequence again while leading with the opposite leg. This sequence dovetails nicely with lesson two's sequence, so once you feel comfortable with these new poses you can do a longer yoga practice by combining all of the sequences we have learned so far.

STANDING SEQUENCE OVERVIEW

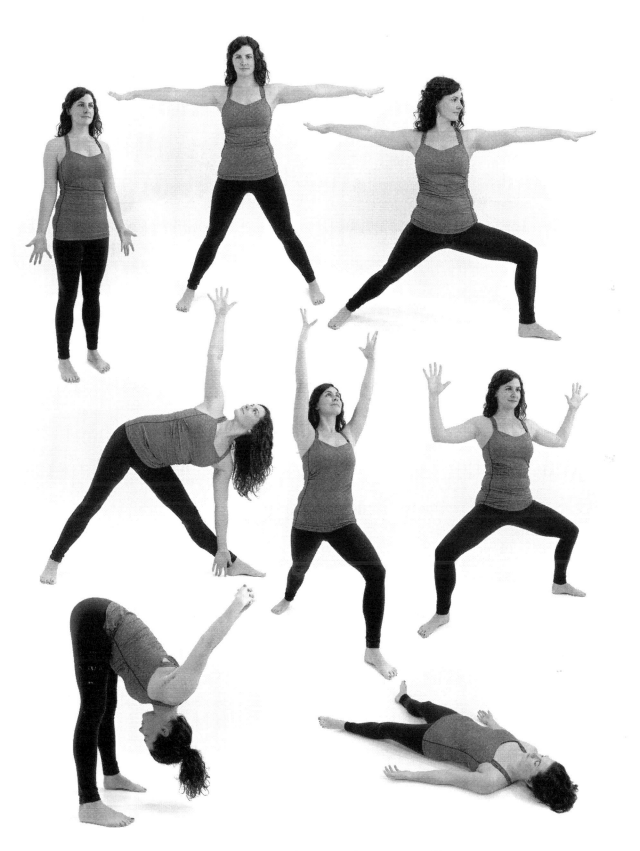

Five-Pointed Star or Trikonasana

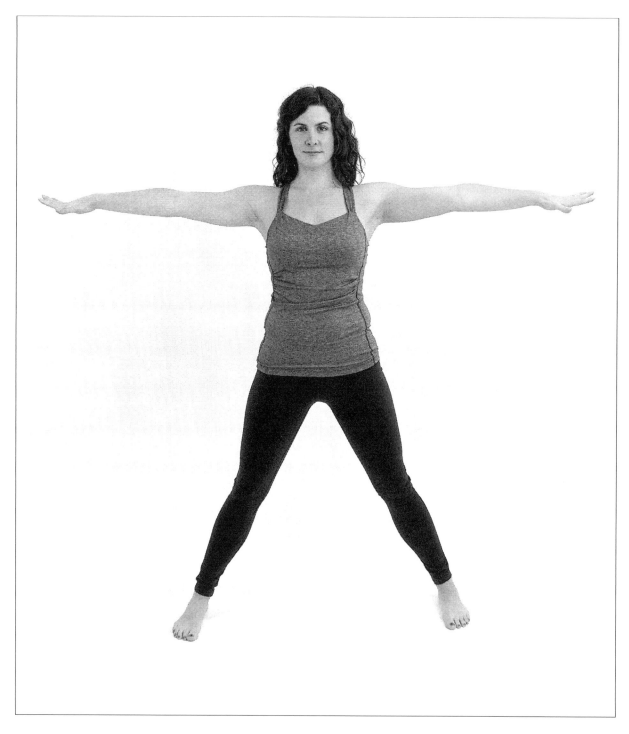

This is a great preparatory pose for all of the standing lunging poses. The simplicity of the alignment of this pose allows you to really feel how to expand and radiate outwards through being grounded in the legs.

Instructions

1. From mountain pose, step the feet wide apart (about four feet) with the arms out to the side. The feet should be under the wrists, facing forward and parallel.

2. Press your weight evenly into the feet, pull up the knee caps, and hug the legs slightly towards each other. Hug the navel and tailbone towards each other, and feel the legs strong and solid, rooted into the floor.

3. Inhale and reach out through the fingertips towards the side walls. Relax the shoulders down and back, very slightly reach the arms to the wall behind you, and reach the sternum forward to gently open the chest.

4. Inhale and reach the crown of the head up to lengthen the spine. Look straight ahead with the chin parallel to the floor.

5. Keep breathing and hold for 2-6 breaths, feeling your body expanding out in five directions.

6. To release, bend one knee and step back into mountain pose.

Benefits: Five-pointed star lengthens, opens, and energizes the whole body. This posture also opens the chest, improving circulation and respiration.

Modifications: Place the hands on the hips.

Warrior II or Virabhadrasana II

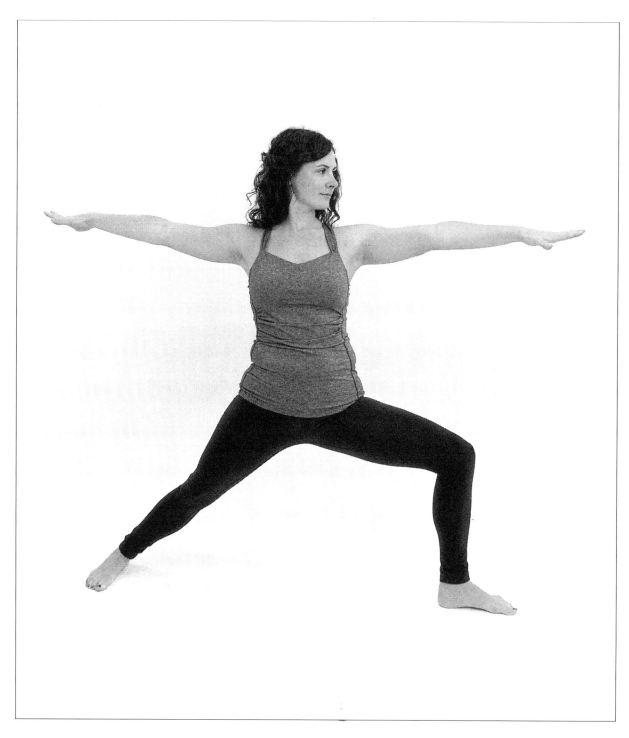

You can embody the focus, determination, and power of this warrior pose through the intensity of your gaze and the muscular activation in your legs. Use this warrior power to stare down any personal problems with the conviction and confidence to conquer and overcome them.

Instructions

1. From a standing position with the legs about four feet apart as in five-pointed star, turn the right toes to the right wall, and bend the right knee over the right ankle with the knee pointing directly at the toes.

2. Turn the hips and the shoulders away from the bent knee, press into the pinky toes sides of the feet, feeling the strong external rotation of the thighs. Inhale and reach out through the finger tips, and turn and look at the right middle finger.

3. Hug the legs towards each other to feel them strong and grounded while you reach up through the crown of the head to lengthen the spine. Relax the shoulders down and back, pressing the chest forward.

4. Breathe and hold for 3-6 breaths.

5. To release, straighten the legs and turn the feet forward coming back into five-pointed star.

6. Repeat on the other side.

Benefits: Warrior II strengthens the legs and opens the hips and chest. Warrior II develops concentration, balance, and groundedness. This pose also improves circulation and respiration, and energizes the entire body.

Contraindications: Recent or chronic injury to the hips, knees or shoulders.

Modifications: A) Place hands on hips. B) Turn palms to face up

Triangle or Utthita Trikonasana

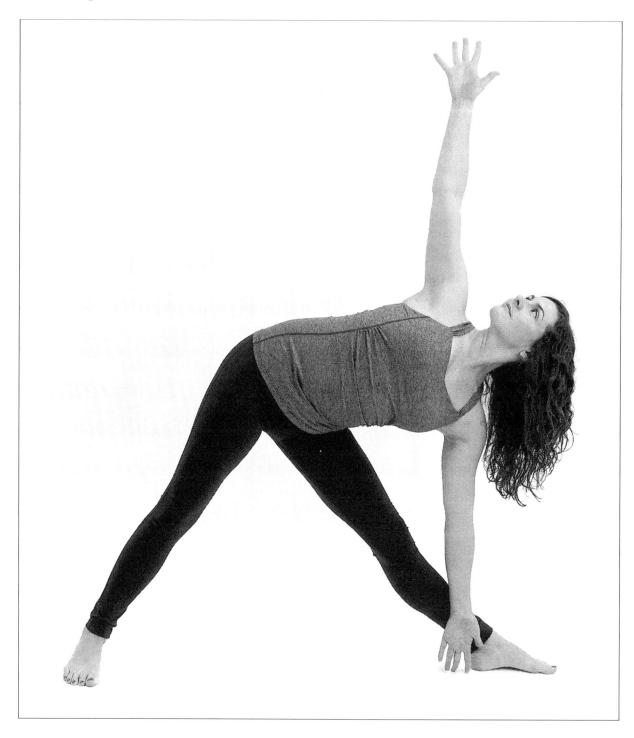

I tell my students to feel the arms, legs and spine long and straight like a triangle in this pose. Pay special attention to keeping the front leg as straight as possible in triangle pose.

Instructions

1. From a standing position with the legs about four feet apart as in five-pointed star, turn the right toes to the right wall and the left toes slightly inwards. Inhale and press the left hips out to the left as you slide both arms to the right, parallel to the floor.

2. Exhale and rotate the arms, reaching the left arm up and resting the right hand against the right leg or down to the floor with the palms facing forward. Have as little weight as possible in the lower hand to encourage your core strength to support you.

3. Press into the feet, and hug the legs towards each other, feeling them strong. Reach the finger tips away from each other, bringing the arms into one straight line with the shoulders stacked on top of each other. Lean the head, shoulders, and arms back so they are directly over the legs, and gaze up towards the left fingertips.

4. Breathe and hold for 3-6 breaths.

5. To release, inhale and reach the raised hand up towards the ceiling as you press down into the feet using the whole body to lift back into five-Pointed Star.

6. Repeat on the other side.

Benefits: Triangle pose engages every part of the body, strengthens the core, opens the hips and shoulders, and stretches the legs.

Contraindications: Recent or chronic injury to the hips, back or shoulders.

Modifications: A) Use a yoga block on the floor to support the lower hand. B) Practice against a wall, leaning the arms, hips, shoulders and head back against the wall for support.

Variations: A) Bring the raised arm over the ear and parallel to the floor. B) The lower hand can rest on the floor on the inside or outside of the leg, or the lower hand can grasp the big toe with the middle and index fingers.

Warrior I or Virabhadrasana I

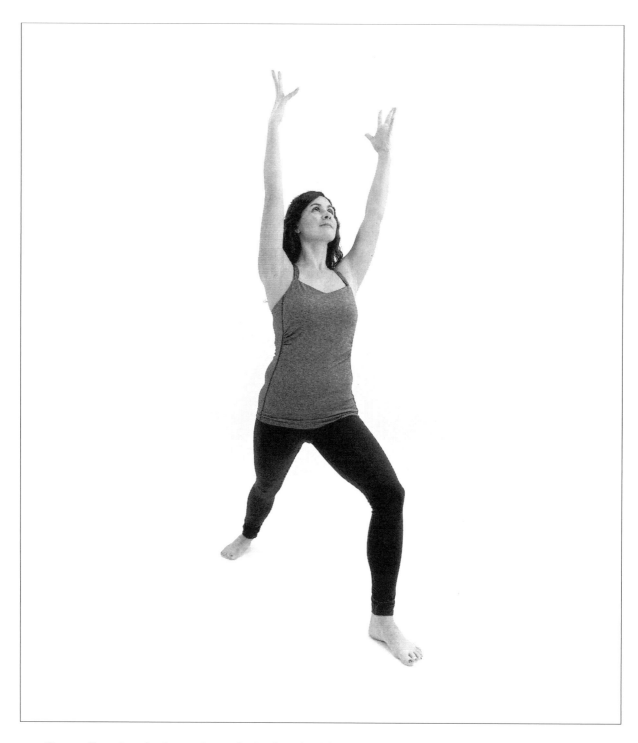

Grounding deeply down through the legs in this posture will support you to lift your heart and gaze up high to embody the brave, victorious and confidant energy of the warrior.

Instructions

1. From a standing position with the legs about four feet apart as in five-pointed star, turn the right toes to the right wall, and bend the right knee over the right ankle with the knee pointing directly at the toes.

2. Bring the hands to the hips and square the hips and the shoulders towards the bent knee. Turn the back foot towards the bent knee to help square the hips forward. Press evenly into both feet, and hug the legs slightly towards each other for more stability.

3. Inhale the arms over the head in an H position with the palms facing each other, bring the palms together crossing the thumbs, or interlace the fingers together and point the index finger up. Modify the position of the arms to keep the shoulders relaxed.

4. Arching your spine, reach the thumbs towards the wall behind you, and lift the heart and the gaze up high.

5. Keep breathing and hold for 3-6 breaths.

6. To release, straighten the legs and turn the feet forward coming back into five-pointed star.

7. Repeat on the other side.

Benefits: Warrior I strengthens the legs, opens the hips and chest, and stretches the arms and legs. Warrior I develops concentration, balance, and groundedness. This pose also improves circulation and respiration and energizes the entire body.

Contraindications: Recent or chronic injury to the hips, knees, back or shoulders.

Modifications: Have the elbows bent in a cactus shape or the arms in a "Y" shape to reduce shoulder tension.

Goddess Squat or Utkata Konasana

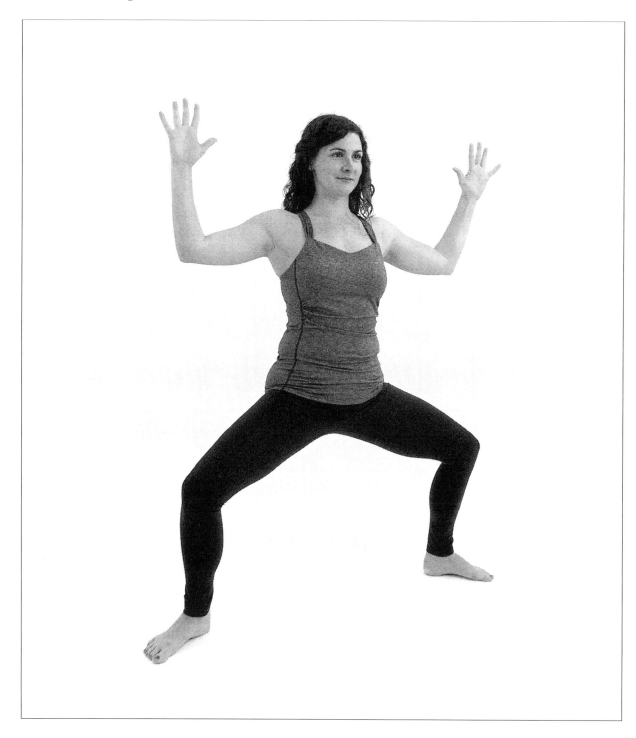

This deep, powerful squatting pose will strengthen the legs and help you cultivate abhyasa, right effort and willful action.

Instructions

1. From a standing position with the feet about three feet apart, bend the elbows at shoulder height, and turn the palms facing each other. Turn the feet out 45 degrees facing the corners of the room, and as you exhale, bend the knees over the ankles squatting down.

2. Press the hips forward, and reach the knees back. Drop the shoulders down and back, and press the chest toward the front of the room. Keep the arms active, with the elbows reaching away from you and with the fingers lightly spreading apart.

3. Breathe and hold for 3-6 breaths.

4. To release, inhale and straighten the legs, reaching the fingertips to the ceiling, then exhale the arms to the sides.

Benefits: Goddess squat pose opens the hips and chest while strengthening and toning the lower body.

Contraindications: Recent or chronic injury to the knees, hips or shoulders.

Standing Yoga Mudra or Dandayamana Yoga Mudrasana

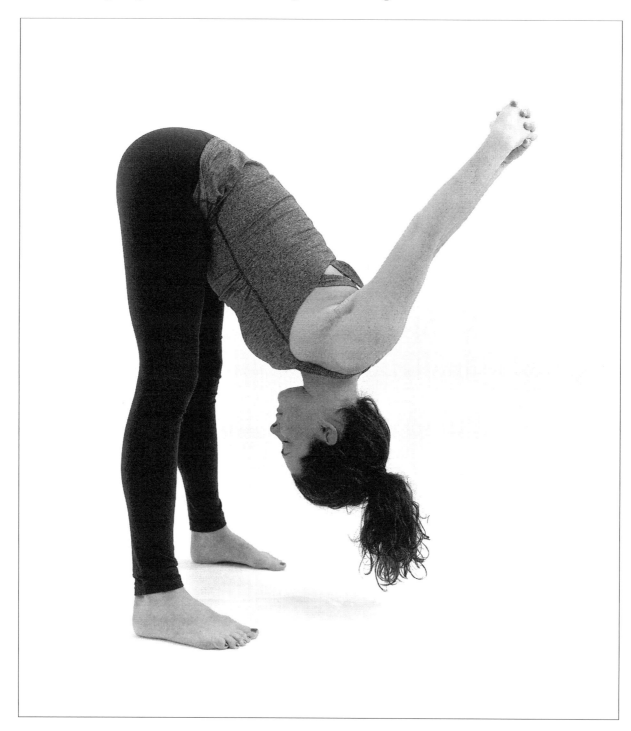

The deep opening through the chest and lungs is unique to this forward bending pose. It is also a great pose to both strengthen and stretch the muscles around the shoulders.

Instructions

1. From a standing position with the legs about four feet apart as in five-pointed star, interlace your fingers behind your back. Inhale and draw the shoulder blades towards each other, and lift the chest and gaze up towards the ceiling.

2. Exhale and hinge at the hips, coming forward with the chest, and reaching the arms up and forward. Let the head relax from the neck, and reach the arms up and forward.

3. Keep the arms and legs straight, and breathe deeply into the belly and chest. If you feel the weight back in the heels, try and shift your weight forward slightly.

4. Breathe and hold for 4-8 breaths.

5. To release, keep the shoulder blades squeezed together as you inhale back up, taking a deep breath into the belly and chest. Exhale and release the arms.

Benefits: Standing yoga mudra improves mental functions, harmonizes the connection between the heart and mind, opens the shoulders, and stretches the upper back and legs.

Contraindications: Unmedicated high blood pressure, recent or chronic injury to the legs, back, neck or shoulders.

Modifications: A) Hold a yoga strap between the hands. B) Step the feet wider apart to make the pose easier, step them closer to make it more challenging.

Drawing Inwards & Twisting Upwards

PRATYAHARA: INWARD FOCUS

In this lesson we will learn how to draw our attention inwards through the yogic technique of Pratyahara, which translates as "gaining mastery over external influences." This is a technique to turn off the external world of sensation and tune into the inner world of the breath and the body's sensations. The analogy that best illuminates this idea is the image of a turtle withdrawing its limbs into its shell — the turtle's shell is the body and mind and the sense organs are the turtle's limbs and head.

By withdrawing our attention from the external sense organs and by focusing inwards on the breath and internal sensations, we still the mind and increase our awareness of the body. With this awareness and focus, we can move deeper into our experience of yoga, as well as harness the energy that is wasted when our minds are distracted by and reacting to external sensations.

There are several different methods to practicing pratyahara; the three easiest are to create a nurturing and supportive practice environment, to close the eyes while practicing, and to create visualizations. By creating a calming environment, you can reduce the external distractions and minimize the power of the external environment to draw on your senses. Surround yourself with soft colors, dim lighting (try burning candles), create a quiet space (turn off phone) or use soft calming music, and most importantly, practice in a clean, uncluttered space. When practicing the yoga poses, it is helpful to first have the eyes open to make sure that you are in the pose properly and that your physical alignment is correct. Once you have attained the physical alignment of the pose, close your eyes and bring your focus and awareness inward to the breath and sensations arising from the body. Another simple way to practice pratyahara is to use visualizations, which create a positive inner impression in the mind. Visualize the look and feel of the pose as you are working and moving deeper into it. Even if you cannot achieve the full expression of the pose, visualizing your body in the full expression will guide you deeper into the pose with more focus and concentration.

SPIRALING UPWARDS

As we learned in Lesson 1, creating the greatest range of movement in the spine relies on our ability to axially lengthen the spine prior to the six movements of the spine. This concept applies most specifically to the twisting poses that we will be learning in this lesson. When moving into a twisting pose, always lengthen the spine on an inhalation and then rotate into the twist on the exhalation. Even when you are holding the twisting pose.

you can continue this action in a subtle way, inhaling and lengthening in the spine and exhaling to rotate a bit deeper into the twist.

Twists have a unique action on the torso, squeezing and compressing the internal organs to flush out toxins, metabolic wastes, and de-oxygenated blood in the same way that wringing out a wet towel squeezes out dirty water. When the twist is released, a fresh supply of blood flows into these areas, carrying oxygen and the building blocks for tissue healing and regeneration. This compression action on the internal organs also massages and tones them, keeping them healthy and strong.

Twisting yoga poses are beneficial for the spine and the muscles surrounding the spine. Twisting poses strengthen the muscles that connect each vertebra, as well as stretching them to facilitate a strong, yet flexible, spine.

While twisting poses are beneficial to the spine and internal organs, never force or torque yourself into the twist with your arms or shoulders. Try to find the perfect balance of using your abdominal and core muscles with the pulling action of the arms. And always think of "twisting upwards" – lengthening first and then twisting – to create the maximum twist when we practice the twisting poses in this lesson's practice session.

PRACTICE SESSION: TWISTING POSES

In this practice session, we will be exploring the most common twisting poses. I find the twisting poses to be some of the most delicious poses in yoga, and I hope you enjoy the wonderful stretch these poses create through the back muscles. Experiment and play with the different techniques of pratyahara to draw your focus inwards in these poses.

This practice session is very similar to the foundational sequence in lesson two, so it can be easily combined with lesson three's sequence for a longer and more challenging practice. You can also add in the previously learned poses in lesson two to make it a bit longer. Please start your practice with the warm-up sequence we learned in the first lesson, and practice Dirga Pranayama at the beginning and/or end of this lesson.

TWISTING SEQUENCE OVERVIEW

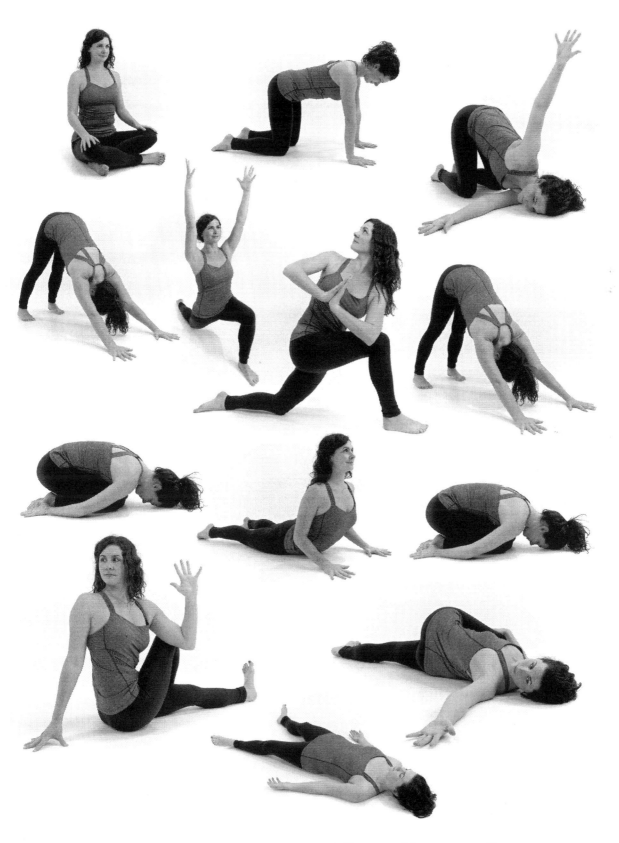

Threading The Needle or Sucirandhrasana

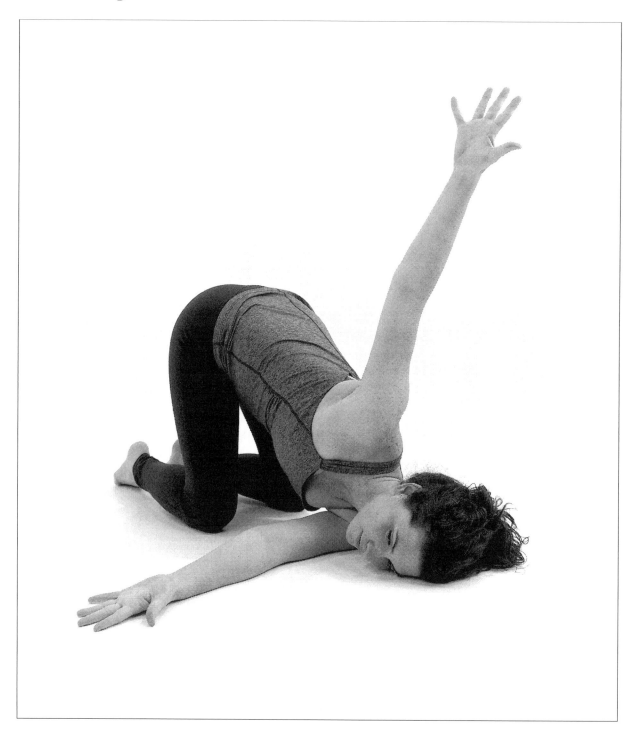

This is a wonderful upper body twist, but it can be a bit awkward to get into the pose. Make sure you have the lower shoulder carefully placed as the foundation for this pose — often the first "landing" of the shoulder is a bit off.

Instructions

1. Come onto you hands and knees as in table pose. Inhale and reach the right hand up towards the ceiling. Exhale and slide the right hand between the left hand and left knee. Slide the arm all the way out to the left so that the right shoulder and side of the head rest comfortably on the floor.

2. Inhale and reach the left hand up towards the ceiling. At first, explore the posture with the raised arm, finding the place were you feel the deepest stretch, then stay there and reach out through the fingers.

3. Breathe and hold for 3-6 breaths.

4. To release, exhale the palm back to the floor, and slowly inhale back to Table pose.

5. Repeat on the other side.

Benefits: Threading the needle pose stretches the shoulders, arms, upper back and neck.

Contraindications: Recent or chronic injury to the knees, shoulders, or neck.

Modifications: Place a folded blanket under the knees to protect them from pressure and stress.

Variations: Cross upper hand over back and hold onto the inside of opposite thigh.

Half Prayer Twist or Ardha Namaskar Parsvakonasana

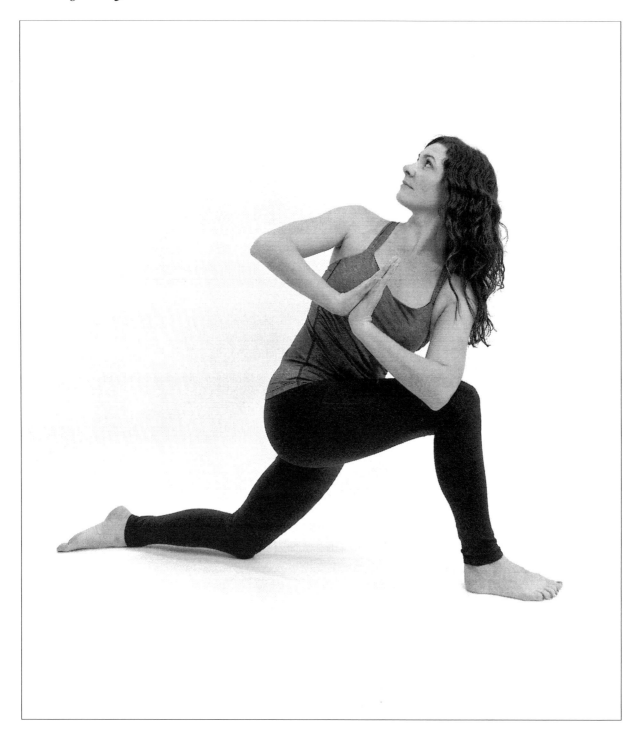

This is a challenging twisting pose, but don't compromise your foundation in the legs to twist through the upper back. Remember to keep the prayer part of the pose; draw your focus to the heart as you reach the thumbs and sternum towards each other.

Instructions

1. From table position, step the right foot between the hands, bringing the right knee directly over the right ankle in a low lunge. The left knee and foot rests on the floor.

2. Bring the left elbow to the right knee and place the palms together in a prayer position. Use the arms to press the right shoulder up and back, twisting the upper back.

3. Look straight ahead or up towards the ceiling. The palms are at the center of the chest and the fingers are pointing up towards the throat. Lift the ribs away from the thigh, and reach out through the crown of the head to avoid collapsing into the pose.

4. Breathe and hold for 4-8 breaths.

5. To release, exhale the arms back down to the floor in a low lunge position.

6. Repeat on the other side.

Benefits: Half prayer twist opens the chest and hips, stretches the back muscles, and nourishes and realigns the spine.

Contraindications: Recent or chronic injury to the hips, knees, back or shoulders.

Modifications: Place a folded blanket under the knees to protect them from excess pressure.

Variations: A) Open the arms wide if you want more stretch in the arms and shoulders. B) Half prayer twist is a an easier variation of prayer twist. If you wish to deepen the pose into the full variation, tuck the toes under, lift the back knee off the floor, and straighten the back leg.

Seated Twist or Ardha Matsyendrasana

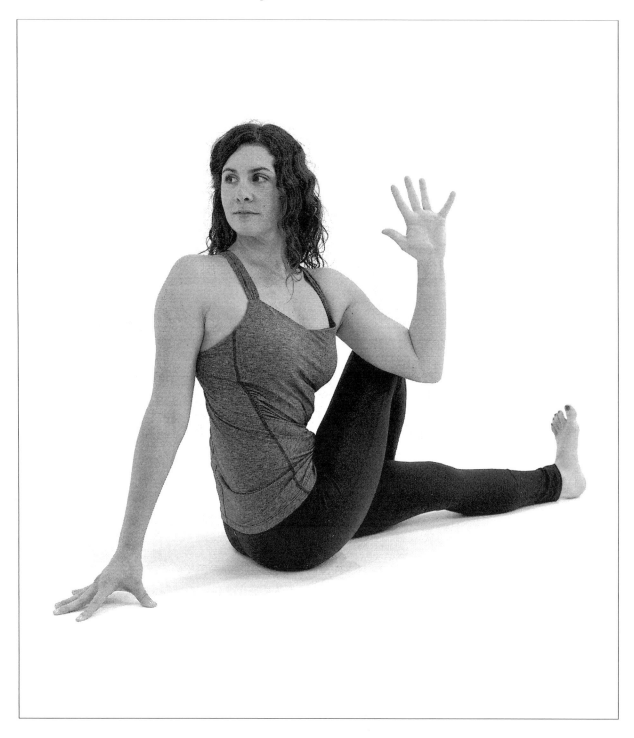

Several of the twisting poses are named after sages or Hindu deities. This seated twist is named after the the great yogi, Matsyendranath, considered by some to be a founding father of modern yoga.

Instructions

1. From a seated position, extend the right leg straight out in front of you. While bending the left knee, cross the left leg over the right, placing the left foot flat on the floor close to the right knee.

2. Wrap the right arm around the left knee and hug the knee in towards your chest. Press down evenly through the sitting bones, and reach up through the crown to lengthen the spine.

3. Inhale and reach the left hand up to lengthen even more. Exhale the arm behind your back placing the palm or fingers on the floor. Look over the left shoulder towards the back wall. For a deeper twist, place the right elbow to the inside of the left knee.

4. As you inhale, press the hips down and reach the crown up to lengthen the spine. As you exhale use the arms to gently deepen the twist. Relax the shoulders down, and press the chest open.

5. Breathe and hold for 4-7 breaths.

6. To release, inhale the left hand up and exhale, untwisting the body, facing the front.

7. Repeat on the other side.

Benefits: Half lord of the fishes pose opens, lengthens, nourishes and realigns the spine. This pose stimulates the nervous, digestive and reproductive systems.

Contraindications: Recent or chronic hip, back or shoulder injury or inflammation.

Modifications: Place a yoga block under the hand behind your back.

Knee Down Twist or Supta Matsyendrasana

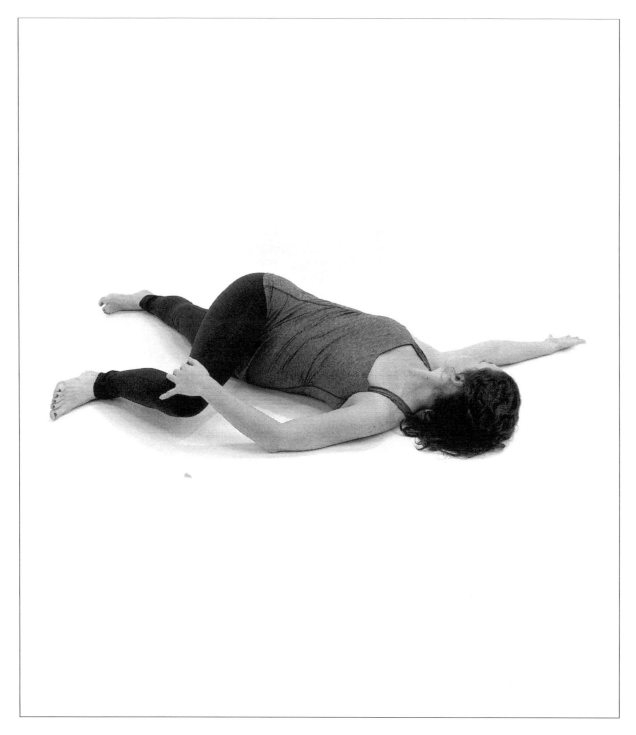

To fully soak up and savor the sweetness of this deep stretch to the back muscles, let this twisting pose be completely effortless.

Instructions

1. Lying on your back, bring your arms out to the sides in a "T" position, palms facing up or down. Bend the right knee and place the right foot on the left knee.

2. Exhale, and drop the right knee over to the left side of your body, twisting the spine and low back. Look back at the right finger tips.

3. Keep the shoulders flat to the floor, close the eyes, and relax into the posture. Let gravity pull the knee down so you do not have to use any effort in this posture. For a deeper twist, bring the bent knee up closer to your shoulder.

4. Breathe and hold for 6-8 breaths.

5. To release, inhale and roll the hips back to the floor. Then exhale the leg back down to the floor.

6. Repeat on other side.

Benefits: Knee down twist stretches the back muscles, realigns and lengthens the spine, and hydrates the spinal disks.

Contraindications: Recent or chronic injury to the knees, hips or back.

Modifications: Place a folded blanket under the bent knee to support it.

Variations: Rest the left hand on the bent knee, adding more weight for gravity to gently pull the knee down.

The Yoga Scientist

SWADYAYA: SELF-OBSERVATION & SELF-INQUIRY

The practice of yoga is often referred to as a science of personal inquiry. While yogic techniques have been developed over many centuries by millions of yogis, students must practice in order to determine if these yogic concepts, philosophies, and practices are appropriate for them. To be able to know if something works, students need to practice Swadyaya, which translates as "self-study." Swadyaya is the ability to observe and witness your thoughts, feelings, emotions and sensations as separate from your Self.

Consciously witnessing what arises within is essential to creating objectivity, without which we lose our discernment or ability to judge if the yoga practices work and ring true to us. There are many different terms describing how to achieve swadyaya, including self-observation, self-inquiry, and mindfulness, but overall, the technique of swadyaya is simple: step back and observe yourself. However, the practice is difficult and requires constancy and diligence since the mind is endlessly fascinated with its own projections, creations, and thoughts.

An easy way to begin practicing swadyaya is to ask yourself one or more inquiry questions while practicing yoga. In this lesson's new poses I've listed a specific inquiry question to help direct your attention inwards and encourage you to observe what is happening. Here are a few general example questions you can practice in any yoga pose:

- How can I be more present in this moment?
- How is this yoga pose different than the last?
- How can I deepen my experience in this moment?
- Am I breathing slowly and deeply in this pose?

Playing the role of the witnessing yoga scientist not only gives us the ability to validate yogic techniques and practices, but allows us to uncover and transcend our ingrained and unconscious thoughts, behaviors, and patterns. When we take swadyaya to this depth, it is important to be compassionate and have an open and accepting attitude towards ourselves and our limitations.

FORWARD BENDING

In this lesson, we will learn several forward-bending poses. Forward bends are known for their innate ability to draw our focus inwards, to calm the body, quiet the mind, and relieve anxiety. Forward bends stretch the backs of the legs (hamstrings and calves) as well stretch the muscles of the back. Many forward bends also compress the abdomen, promoting the total exhalation of air from the lungs, and strengthening the muscles of respiration.

Many of the forward bending poses cause the back to round which, in turn, stretches the muscles in the back and compresses the front of the spine. This rounding of the back can aggravate chronic and acute conditions such as back strain and herniated discs. Therefore, these poses should be avoided or approached with caution in these conditions.

The safest way to move into a forward-bending pose is to lengthen the spine first, then hinge forward from the hips, and lastly, round the spine forward. Remember to practice ahimsa (non-harming), and try to not push or pull yourself past your edge in these poses. If you have concerns with your back, you can hold the pose with a flat back instead. We will go over how to move into the forward bends in detail in this lesson's practice session.

PRACTICE SESSION: FORWARD BENDS

Swadyaya builds on the previous lesson's practice of pratyahara, looking inwards. In this practice session, work towards detaching yourself from the experience, and try to create a sense of witnessing the pose. Use each posture as an opportunity to play scientist and learn about your body, mind, and spirit. Notice what thoughts, reactions, and responses are created in each pose, and question these patterns by asking "why am I thinking, feeling, or reacting this way in this pose?"

This practice session can be easily combined with lesson three's sequence for a longer and more challenging practice. You can also add in any of the previously learned poses to make it longer. Please start your practice with the warm-up sequence we learned in the first lesson, and practice dirga pranayama at the beginning and/or end of this lesson.

FORWARD BENDING SEQUENCE OVERVIEW

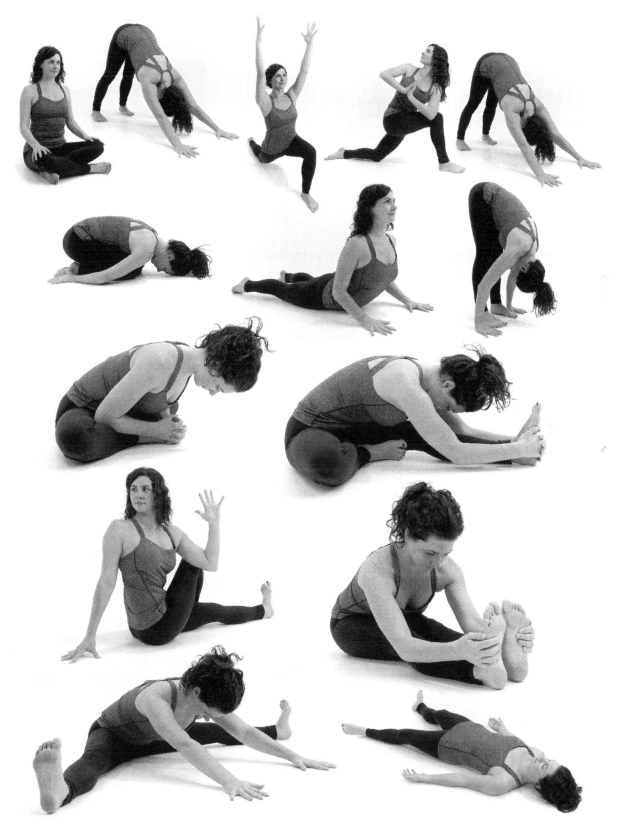

Bound Angle or Baddha Konasana

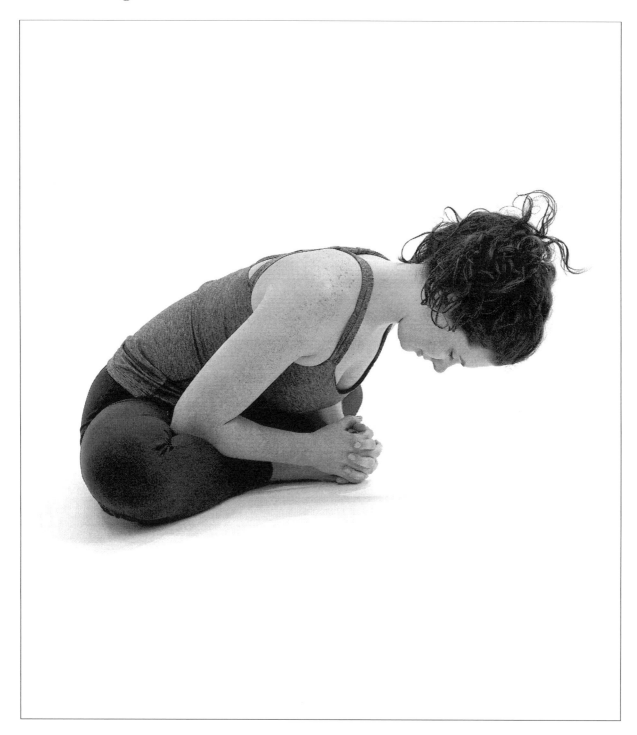

This is my favorite hip opening pose. Bound angle is one of the easiest and gentlest poses to stretch the groin and open the hips. What insights arise as you gaze at the third eye point in this pose?

Instructions

1. From a seated position, bring the bottoms of the feet together with the knees bent out to the sides, and interlace the fingers around the toes, or hold onto the ankles.

2. Inhale, press the sitting bones down, and reach the crown of the head up towards the ceiling. Exhale and relax the shoulders down and back; inhale and press the chest towards the front. With the eyes open or closed, gaze up at the third eye point.

3. Exhale and gently pull your torso forward. Keep the back flat or round forward, reaching the head towards the toes. If you want more stretch in the hips, gently press the elbows against the legs.

4. Breathe and hold for 3-8 breaths.

Benefits: Bound angle opens the hips and chest, lengthens the spine, and stimulates the reproductive, nervous, and respiratory systems.

Contraindications: Recent or chronic knee or hip injury or inflammation.

Modifications: A) Place a folded blanket under the sitting bones. B) Place folded blankets under the knees.

Variations: Slide the feet 1-2 feet forward, bring the arms under the ankles, and interlace the fingers around the toes. Round forward, pulling the forehead towards the toes with the arms.

Seated Head to Knee or Janu Sirsasana

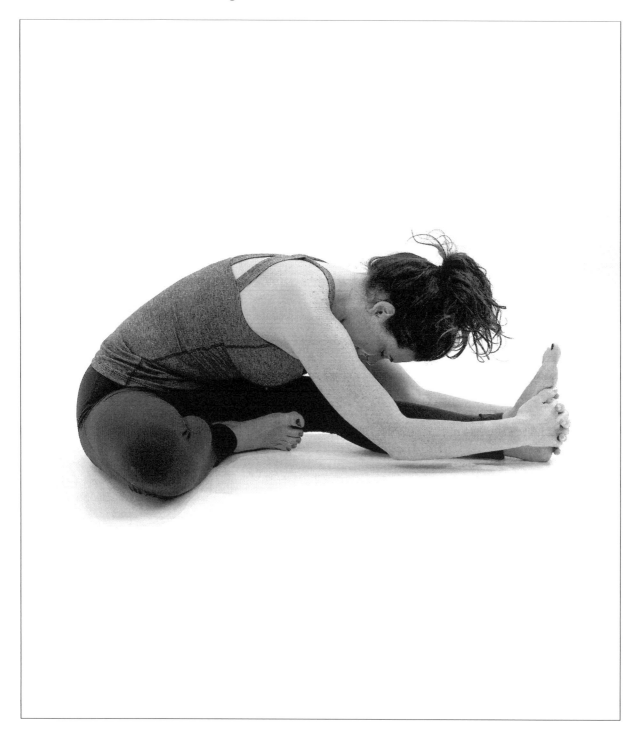

This is a wonderful pose to deeply stretch the hamstrings and to promote a deep sense of peace and calm. Can you trace the lines of stretch from the hip to the toes?

Instructions

1. From a seated position like bound angle or easy pose, extend the right leg straight out in front of you, place the bottom of the left foot against the right thigh. Pull the right leg in to square the hips to the front wall.

2. Inhale the arms up, and reach out of the waist, lengthening the spine.

3. Imagine someone lightly pulling on your fingers as you exhale forward, and let the hands come down to the foot or ankle. The back can stay flat, or you can round and reach the head towards the knee.

4. To deepen the stretch in the hamstrings, gently straighten the extended leg, press out through the heel, and draw the toes towards you using the muscles in the leg. If the back is flat, use the arms to pull the sternum forward. If rounding the back let the head, neck and shoulders completely relax.

5. Breathe and hold for 3-6 breaths.

6. To release, inhale the arms up over your head; exhale them to the floor, or slowly roll up the spine on the inhalation.

7. Repeat on the other side.

Benefits: Seated head to knee stretches the back and deeply stretches the back of the legs. This posture calms the mind and emotions and stimulates the nervous, digestive and endocrine systems.

Cautions: Recent or chronic back or knee injury or inflammation.

Modifications: A) Use a yoga strap around foot of the straight leg, and hold with both hands. B) Use a blanket under the bent knee to reduce straining the knee joint.

Variations: If you have the flexibility, reach the hands in front of the foot, clasping hand to wrist.

Seated Forward Bend or Paschimottanasana

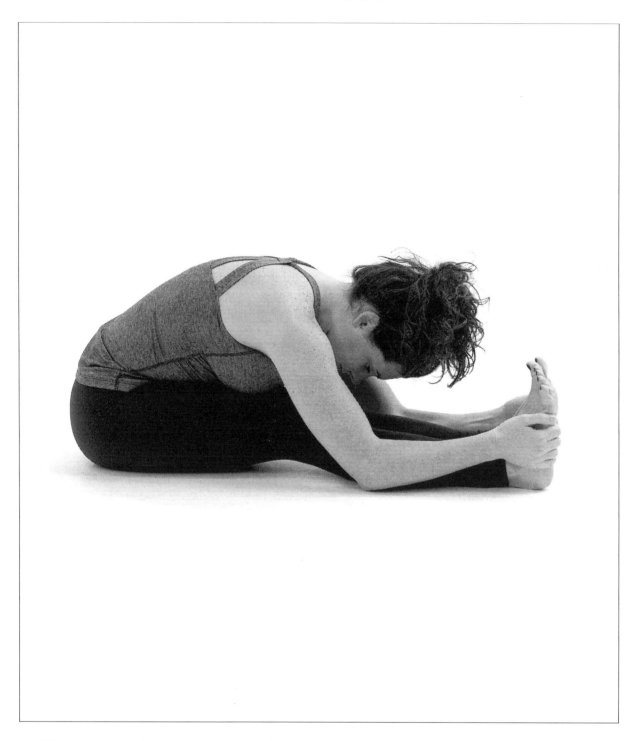

Turn your gaze inwards in this deep forward-bending pose. Where do you feel the deep sense of calm and peace this pose invokes?

Instructions

1. From a seated position with the legs forward and together, inhale the arms up over the head, and lift and lengthen up through the fingers and crown of the head. Relax the shoulders away from the ears, and ground the sitting bones into the floor.

2. Imagine someone lightly pulling on your fingers as you exhale and hinge forward at the hips. Let the hands come down on the toes, ankles, or shins. Keep the back flat or round, and reach the head towards the knees. The knees can be slightly bent.

3. To deepen the stretch in the hamstrings, gently straighten the legs, press out through the heels, and draw the toes towards you using the muscles in the legs. If the back is flat, use the arms to pull the sternum forward. If rounding the back, let the head, neck and shoulders completely relax.

4. Breathe and hold for 3-8 breaths.

5. To release, slowly roll the spine up and back into a seated position.

Benefits: Seated forward fold provides a deep stretch for entire back side of the body from the heels to the neck. Forward Fold calms the nervous system and emotions and stimulates the reproductive and urinary systems.

Contraindications: Recent or chronic injury to the arms, hips, ankles or shoulders.

Modifications: Use a yoga strap around the feet, and hold on to the strap with both hands.

Variations: If you have the flexibility, reach the hands around the feet, clasping hand to wrist.

Seated Angle or Upavistha Konasana

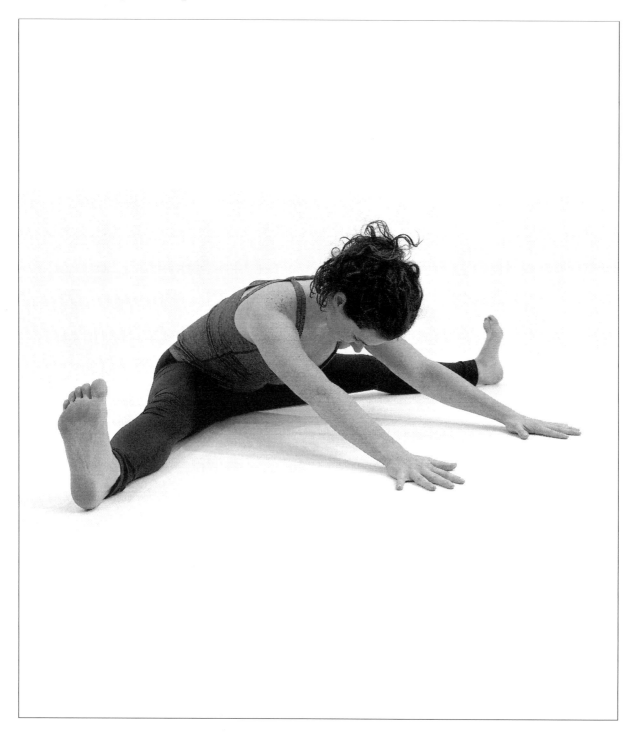

It is easy to feel stuck in this hip opening pose and get caught up in judgment and negative self-talk. Move into this pose slowly with compassion and a focused, witnessing mind. How does your mind react and respond to this challenging forward bend?

Instructions

1. From a seated position with the legs forward, spread the legs out as wide as comfortable with the toes and knee caps pointing straight up.

2. Inhale the arms up towards the ceiling, reach the thumbs to the back wall and the sternum to the front wall. Imagine someone lightly pulling on your fingers as you exhale and hinge forward at the hips. Let the hands come down to the floor, and keep the back flat or round forward.

3. Walk the fingertips forward, or alternatively, you can reach out and hold the ankles or feet to gently deepen the stretch. You can also press out through the heels and reach the toes back to create more stretch in the backs of the legs.

4. Breathe and hold for 3-8 breaths.

5. To release, slowly walk the hands in as you carefully roll up the spine.

Benefits: Seated angle deeply opens the hips while stretching the entire back side of the body.

Contraindications: Recent or chronic injury to the knees, hips, arms or shoulders.

Modifications: A) Place a blanket under the hips or the heels. B) Place a bolster or several blankets between the legs to rest the torso on.

Finding Contentment in Backbends

SANTOSHA: CONTENTMENT

I have found that the progress in yoga is not a steady, continuous path of improvement in flexibility, strength, or ability. There are peaks, plateaus, and dips along the way, which can be frustrating and discouraging, especially to new students. Many beginning students excessively strive to "get there," while others quickly identify the poses that they dislike and avoid them at all cost. These reactions show us how easy it is to become discontent within our practice. If this discontentment is not addressed, then we may needlessly suffer in our practice or end up giving up on yoga altogether.

Santosha (contentment) is considered an essential and fundamental practice in yoga. Practicing contentment frees us from the unnecessary suffering of always wanting things to be different; it encourages us to be present with what is happening and to find the opportunity to learn and grow from our experiences of discontentment. Yoga has taught me that true joy and happiness can only be attained when we are perfectly content with all that life gives us.

Santosha can be practiced while holding yoga poses by letting go of the desire to attain the perfect looking pose and to accept the experience of the pose as it is without wanting to change it. To do this, notice what arises as you move into each pose, and be present with the sensations and feelings without judging or criticizing them. (Judgement, criticism and comparison are the three warning signs that we are not in a state of contentment.) Let go of any attachments of what you think the pose should feel like or look like. When any hint of discontentment arises in the mind, simply let it go and return your focus on the breath and the pure sensations arising in the body. Another strategy to combat discontentment is to invoke feelings of gratitude. (Focus on the simple blessings in your life, being thankful for relationships, something you love to do, your breath, or other physical ability or sensation.) Ultimately, practicing santosha gives us the ability to be at peace in any pose or situation we may find ourselves in, on and off our mats.

BACKBENDS AND COUNTERPOSES

We will be diving into backbends in this lesson's practice session, which can be some of the most intense poses in yoga, but also the most rewarding. Backbends are known to energize, refresh, and invigorate the body and mind. Many backbends also open the chest, lungs, and heart to improve inhalation and receptivity to all of life's challenges. Backbends can elicit fear due to how they dramatically open us outwards, and some require core and back strength to be performed safely (don't worry, we will be only practicing simple and safe ones in this lesson). They are inherently extroverted poses, opening our soft yin or feminine side unprotected outwards towards the external environment.

To counter the fear of bending backwards we must do several things. First we need to be in a safe supportive environment, and we must cultivate an internal focus that can keep our awareness inward as we bend backward. Second, as with all the movements of the spine, we must focus on lengthening the spine before and during a backbend. A common misalignment in backbends is compressing and crunching in the low back or neck. Let your backbends be performed with a long spine and a continuous smooth curve in the back. If you feel any tension in the low back, work on tucking the tailbone under (by tilting the pelvis forward) and/or lengthening the tailbone away from your head to decrease the curve in the low back. Lastly, we need to have a strong back and core to feel safe moving back into a deep backbend. If you feel any strain or discomfort in the low back, then release or soften the effort of the backbend. You can safely build strength in the backbending poses by holding them for shorter times and doing multiple repetitions of the pose.

Our everyday lives require much forward-bending, and we do many activities from a slouched or hunched position. This constant rounding of the spine is nicely balanced through performing backbending poses. But due to the intensity of the backbends, it is always advised to follow them with a forward bending "counterpose" to release any tension created in the low back. Using a counterpose creates balance in the body and spine and calms the mind after the energizing effects of the backbend.

The breath is the "canary in the coal mine" in backbending poses. Make sure that your breath is always slow and deep when moving into and holding the backbends. If you notice that your breath has stopped or feels restricted, you have gone too far into the pose; either ease out of the pose to the point where you can breathe deeply, or come out of the pose completely. Slow, deep breathing helps us to work safely in backbends and to feel calm and less fearful of moving deep into the pose.

PRACTICE SESSION: BACKBENDING

It is easy to feel overwhelmed by the intense strength needed to perform the backbending poses. You can build up to this strength by starting with shorter holds with multiple repetitions of the pose. I tell my students that backbending poses should feel exciting and invigorating. I find focusing on both the stimulating and strengthening effects of these poses helps to bring an easier sense of contentment to them.

For a longer and more challenging practice insert lesson three's standing sequence after the second downward dog. You can also add in any of the previously learned poses to make it longer. Please start your practice with the warm-up sequence we learned in the first lesson, and practice Dirga Pranayama at the beginning and/or end of this lesson.

BACKBENDING SEQUENCE OVERVIEW

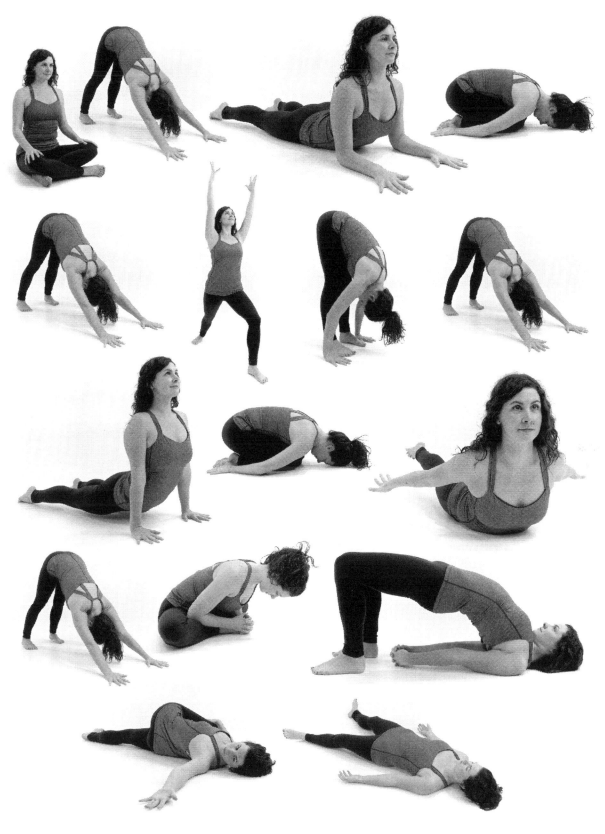

Sphinx or Salamba Bhujangasana

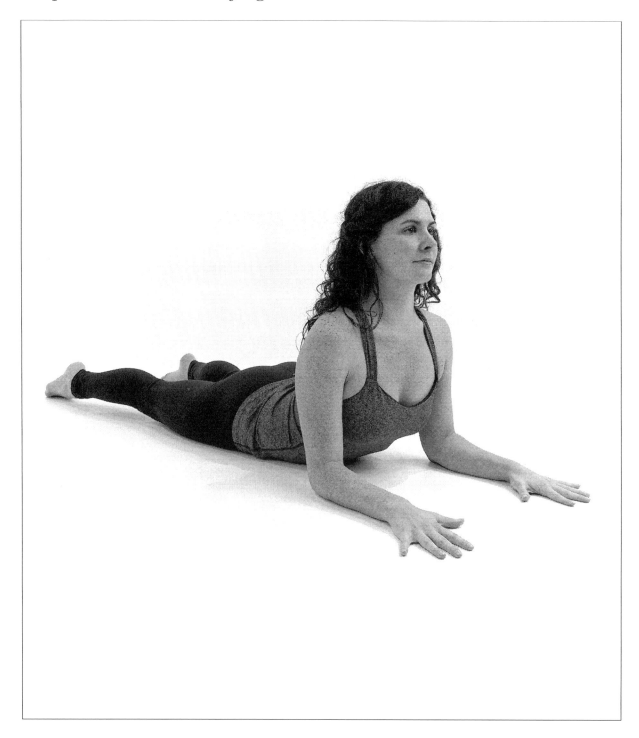

Sphinx is a very gentle backbending pose that deeply opens the chest and ribs. Learning how to use the arms to draw the sternum forward and reach up through the crown of the head in sphinx will be applicable in the several other backbending poses.

Instructions

1. Lie on your belly with the forearms flat on the floor, elbows under the shoulders, to prop up your torso. Have the fingers pointing straight ahead and the legs together.

2. Press the forearms, pubic bone and feet down into the floor. Inhale and lift the head and chest up and back.

3. Keep the elbows close to your sides, and use the arms to lift you up even higher. Relax the shoulders down and back, and use the arms to reach the chest forward. Draw the chin in towards the back of the neck, and gaze up at the third eye point.

4. Breathe and hold for 2-6 breaths.

5. To release, exhale and bend the knees, pressing the hips back to the heels in child's pose.

Benefits: Sphinx opens the chest and strengthens the arms and shoulders. Sphinx aligns the spine and invigorates the kidneys and nervous system.

Contraindications: Recent or chronic injury to the back, arms or shoulders, pregnancy or recent abdominal surgery.

Variations: If you want more challenge, you can lift the elbows an inch or two off the floor.

Upward Facing Dog or Urdhva Mukha Svanasana

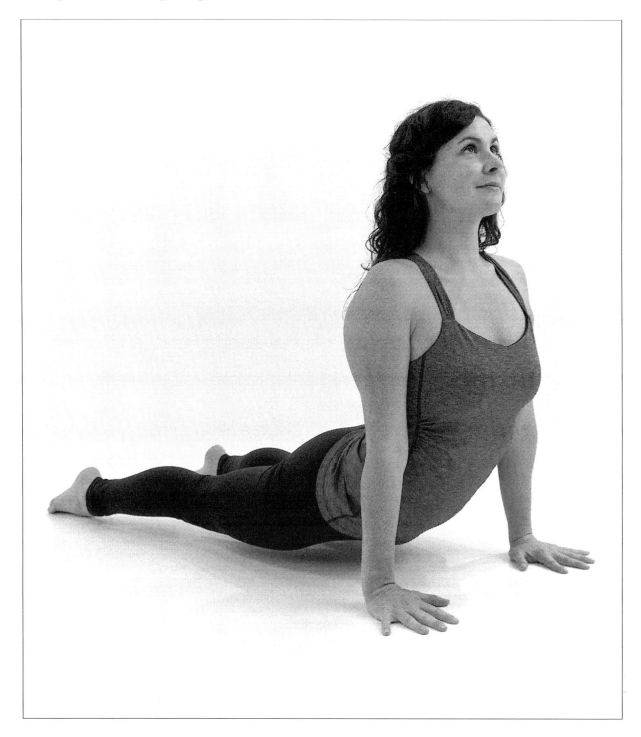

Upward facing dog is similar to the cobra pose that we learned in lesson two but much more challenging. See if you find contentment in this deep opening in the front of the body.

Instructions

1. From table pose, walk the hands one hand length forward, and spread the fingers wide apart. Exhale and slowly drop the hips forward toward the floor.

2. Press out into the fingertips to lift the head and shoulders up and back. Relax the shoulders down and back, reach the chest forward, and press the crown of the head up towards the ceiling.

3. Inhale and lift thighs and legs off of the floor by pressing the tops of the feet down, engaging the thighs, and hugging the legs towards each other.

4. Breathe and hold for 1-3 breaths.

5. To release, bend the knees, and lift the hips back up into table position or bring the hips back to the heels in child's pose.

Benefits: Upward facing dog opens the chest and strengthens the arms, legs and back side of the body. Up dog aligns the spine and invigorates the kidneys and nervous system.

Contraindications: Recent or chronic injury to the back, hips, arms or shoulders, pregnancy and recent abdominal surgery.

Modifications: Place yoga blocks under the palms.

Variations: Have the legs wide apart.

Locust or Shalabhasana

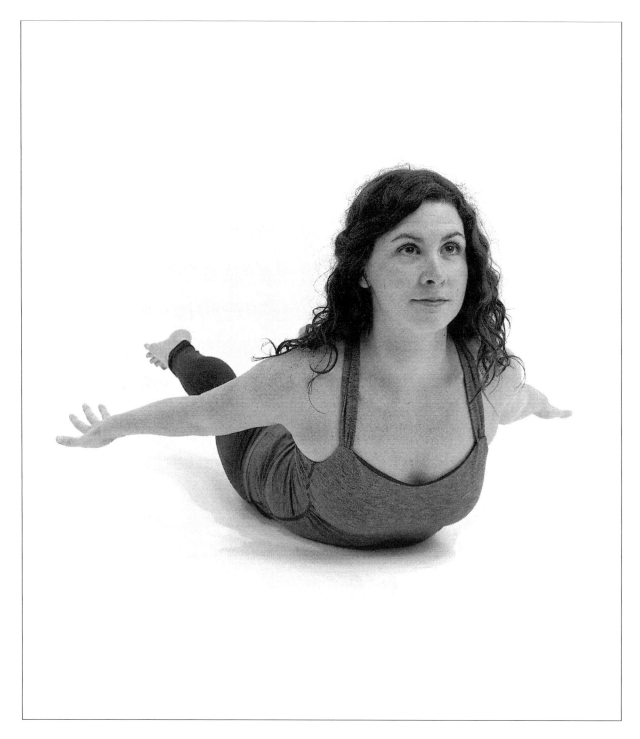

It is easy to get too serious-minded in this intense core strengthening pose. Find contentment in this pose by cultivating a sense of joy and lightheartedness, and see if you can enjoy the intensity of locust.

Instructions

1. Lie on your belly with the chin on the floor, legs together and arms alongside the body, 45 degrees away from the sides with the palms down.

2. Press the pubic bone down into the floor. Inhale and lift the legs, head, chest, and arms off of the floor. Reach out through the fingers, toes, tailbone and crown of the head. Keep the neck in line with the spine.

4. Slide the shoulders towards your waist and reach the sternum forward. Lift your gaze high to your forehead while drawing the chin in towards the center of the neck. Work towards lifting the ribcage off the floor.

5. Breathe and hold for 2-6 breaths.

6. To release, exhale and slowly lower the chest, head, arms and legs to the floor. Turn the head to one side, slide the arms alongside your body and rest. Rock the hips from side to side to release any tension in the low back.

Benefits: Locust pose strengthens the legs and core body while opening the chest and stretching the low back. Locust pose tonifies the kidneys and stimulates the reproductive and digestive systems.

Contraindications: Recent or chronic injury to the back, arms or shoulders, pregnancy, menstruation, or recent abdominal surgery.

Modifications: A) Place a folded blanket under the hips. B) Place a rolled up blanket or bolster under the thighs. C) Place a rolled blanket under the rib cage.

Variations: To make the pose more challenging, bring the arms out to the sides or forward over your head.

Bridge or Setu Bandhasana

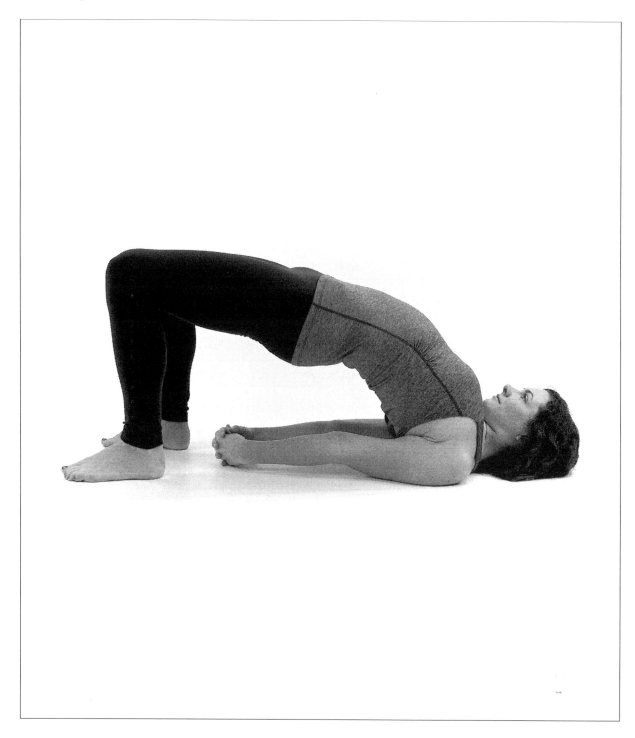

In this deeply energizing backbend, explore how the front of the body needs to open the same amount the back side of the body must engage to lift the torso up high. As you hold this bridge, see if you can be completely present with the build-up and movement of sensations in your body.

Instructions

1. Lying on your back, bend both knees, and place the feet flat on the floor, hip width apart, and directly under your knees. Slide the arms alongside the body with the palms facing down.

2. Press the feet into the floor, inhale and lift the hips up, rolling the spine up to your shoulders. Press a tiny bit more into the big toe sides of the feet to keep the knees pointing straight ahead.

3. If possible, interlace the hands together behind your back, walk the arms and shoulders close together. Press down into the arms and shoulders to lift the chest up. Engage the legs and buttocks to lift the hips higher.

4. If there is discomfort in the low back, reach the tailbone and the knees forward.

5. Breathe and hold for 4-8 breaths.

6. To release, exhale, release the arms and slowly roll the spine back to the floor.

Benefits: Bridge pose builds core and lower body strength, strengthens the spine, energizes the body, and stimulates the endocrine and nervous systems.

Contraindications: Recent or chronic injury to the knees, shoulders or back.

Modifications: A) Use a strap between the hands if you cannot interlace your fingers. B) Use a yoga block under the hips to support your weight.

Concentration and Balance

DHARANA - CONCENTRATION

In Lesson 4, we learned to draw our focus inwards using the practice of pratyahara. In this lesson we will learn how to focus our attention like a laser beam to establish a state of present-mindedness. Dharana (concentration) is a state of complete focused attention on a single object and is the foundation of meditation. Usually we use the body, breath or focal points (drishti) as the object of focus for dharana in a yoga practice since they are easily available. But anything can be used as a point of focus: a visual symbol or figure (mandala or yantra), a symbolic phrase (mantra), or a hand gesture (mudra). We need to just choose a point of focus that works best for us and then work on training our attention to remain fixed on that single point.

When practicing dharana, you will notice how quickly the mind shifts its focus from one thing to the next–thoughts, feelings, memories, and emotions are constantly fluttering through our minds. Whenever you become aware that the mind has become distracted, simply bring it back again to your chosen point of focus without any judgment or disappointment.

At first, this practice of concentration will be difficult, and you may only be able to hold your focus for a few seconds, but each moment of dharana builds upon another. Each time you bring your focus back to dharana, the stronger your will and focus becomes. Practice and patience are essential to strengthen dharana.

The ancient yogis say that there are three enemies of dharana: desire, fear, and boredom. When these states are present, dharana will be especially difficult, so being able to focus on cultivating positive attributes such as contentment, trust, and curiosity before practicing dharana will be helpful.

In this lesson's practice session, we will be working on focusing the mind on the breath and the physical sensations with each posture. We will also be using a drishti (gazing point) as an additional point of focus to use with our yoga practice. Explore these different options with the goal of finding out what type of focal point works best for you.

Drishti - Focal Point

A drishti (view or gaze) is a specific focal point that is employed during meditation or while holding a yoga posture. The ancient yogis discovered that where our gaze is

LESSON SEVEN • CONCENTRATION AND BALANCE   94

directed our attention naturally follows, and that the quality of our gazing is directly reflected in the quality of our mental thoughts. When the gaze is fixed on a single point, the mind is less stimulated by other external objects and can easily enter the state of dharana.

In yoga postures, a drishti is used to guide the direction of the pose, as well as to keep the mind engaged and focused. To use a drishti while in a yoga pose, simply select the point where your gaze is naturally directed by the alignment of the posture. For example, in many of the twisting poses that we practiced in Lesson 4, turning our head and our gaze deepened the twisting action of the pose. The muscles around the eyes should be relaxed, and the gaze should be soft. Do not strain the eyes.

There are eight specific drishtis are used in hatha yoga:

1. Nasagrai Drishti, gaze at the tip of the nose, as used in Locust, Upward Facing Dog and standing forward fold poses.

2. Angusta Ma Dyai Drishti, gaze at the thumbs, as used in Warrior I.

3. Nabi Chakra Drishti, gaze at the navel, as used in Bridge, Downward Facing Dog and most seated forward bends.

4. Pahayoragrai Drishti, gaze at the toes, as used in Upward Boat and Bound Angle.

5. Hastagrai Drishti, gaze at the hands, as used in Triangle and Warrior II.

6. Parsva Drishti, gaze to the side, as used in seated and supine spinal twists.

7. Urdhva Drishti, gaze upwards, as used in Prayer Twist.

8. Naitrayohmadya or **Broomadhya Drishti,** gaze at the third eye or forehead, as used in Chair, Plank, and Upward Forward Fold.

Using a drishti is especially helpful and important during balancing postures. Balancing requires intense mental focus and a calm, centered mind. When our eyes or minds wander, we lose focus and are more likely to fall. In most balance poses the drishti is a point on the floor or wall in front of you.

In bhakti yoga, drishti is used in a slightly different way: a constant loving and longing gaze is turned toward the concept, name or image of the Divine. Drishti can also be thought of in a much broader context: attaining the proper view or perspective of one's life that promotes inner peace and happiness.

BALANCING AND STRENGTHENING POSES

In this practice session we will learn two balancing poses that will require a strong dharana. Our ability to stay balanced in these poses is a direct result of our concentration and ability to stay focused on a drishti point. I've also noticed a relationship between how balanced I feel when practicing these balancing poses and how balanced I am in my life. When something is unbalanced in my life (too much work, not enough sleep, emotional upheaval, etc.), it shows up on my mat as a wobbly pose. You may notice that if you practice balance poses on a regular basis, your ability to balance will shift from day to day. If so, I invite you to see if you can find a similar correlation to physical balance and the overall state of balance in your life.

Additionally, many students compromise grace and form by trying to take the balancing poses to their most advanced expression too quickly. Instead, have the intention of being graceful and humble rather than getting caught by the ego's desire to achieve the highest expression of the pose. If you fall out of the pose, come back to where you were, or come back into an easier variation of the pose. The longer you can maintain your balance in the balancing poses, the stronger your concentration and inner balance will become.

We will also be learning a few strengthening poses that will also challenge our concentration. When we challenge the body on a physical level, the mind will often react to the intense sensations by labeling them as bad, uncomfortable, or torturous. Notice how the mind reacts, but always work toward bringing your focus back to the breath and the sensations in the body. Simply feel the sensations without letting the mind judge them, complain, or criticize. Using a drishti for these poses will be helpful to deepen your dharana and keep you present in the pose.

> "An uncontrolled mind has no wisdom. Without a controlled mind there is no concentration, and without concentration, there can be no tranquility. How can there be happiness chaos rules the mind?"
>
> — Bhagavad Gita

PRACTICE SESSION: BALANCING

Humility and compassion are two essential components for practicing balancing poses. Having a humble attitude will make success easier, and having compassion for yourself will make the struggle with these poses easier to bear. Have the faith to know that, with practice, you will become much better at balancing.

For a longer and more calming practice insert lesson five's sequence after the standing yoga mudra pose. You can also add in any of the previously learned poses to make it longer. Please start your practice with the warm-up sequence we learned in the first lesson, and practice Dirga Pranayama at the beginning and/or end of this lesson.

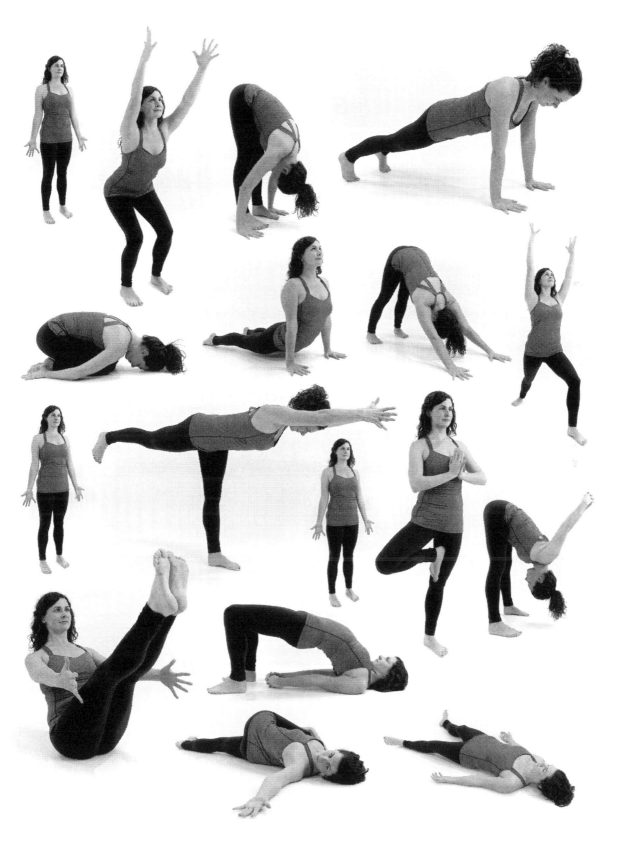

Chair or Utkatasana

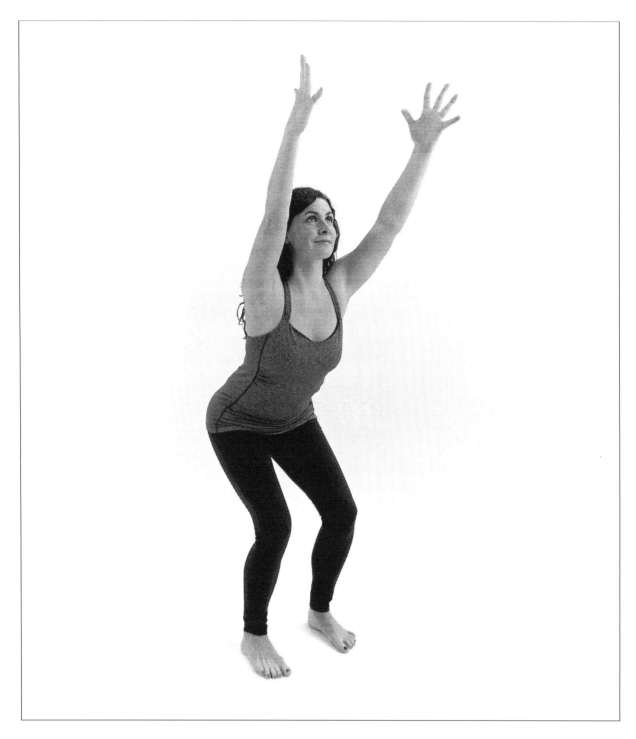

In this "powerful" standing posture, draw the vibrant energy out of pelvis and up into the crown of the head. Let your drishti lift your heart and gaze up high in chair pose.

Instructions

1. In mountain pose with the feet together or hip width apart, exhale and bend the knees, squatting down.

2. Reach the hips down and back as if you were going to sit on the edge of a chair, bringing your weight to the heels of the feet and the knees over the ankles. Do not bring the hips lower than the level of the knees. Make sure that the knees and toes are pointing straight ahead.

3. Relax the shoulders down and back, and reach out through the fingertips. Lift the heart, gaze and fingertips up high.

4. Breathe and hold for 3-6 breaths.

5. To release, inhale and press down into the feet, straightening the legs, and inhale the arms up toward the ceiling. Exhale to release the arms down.

Benefits: Chair pose strengthens the lower body while stretching the upper back. This posture invigorates and energizes the whole body.

Contraindications: Recent or chronic injury to the hips, knees, back or shoulders.

Modifications: Squeeze a yoga block between the thighs to help keep the knees pointing forward.

Variations: To make this pose less challenging, reach the arms forward parallel to the floor or place the hands on the knees.

Plank or Phalakasana

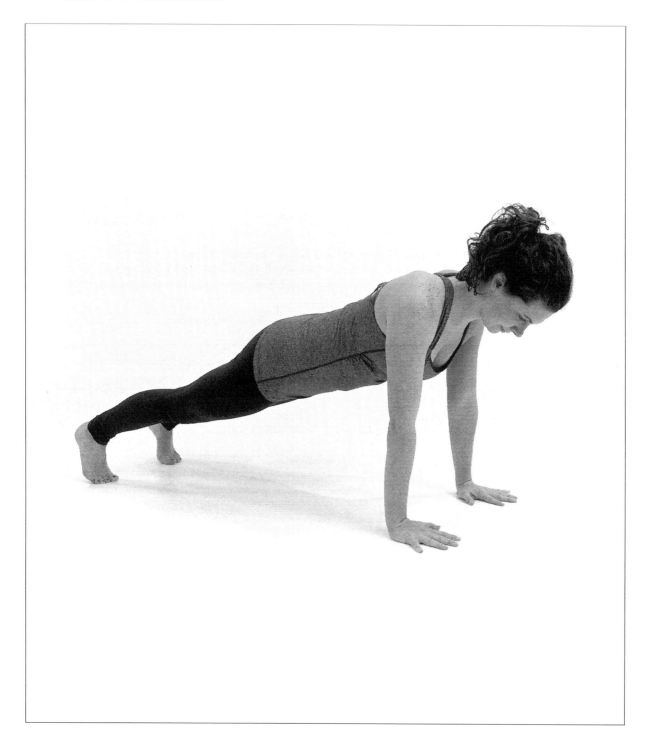

Proper alignment is essential to receive benefits of plank. Let the steadiness of your gaze mirror your steady holding of this intense core-strengthening pose.

Instructions

1. From standing forward fold, step or jump both feet back 4-5 feet into a push-up position.

2. Spread the fingers wide apart with the middle finger pointing forward and the arms straight. Strongly tuck the tailbone under so the legs, hips, and torso are one straight line. Press into the fingertips and knuckles to keep weight out of the wrists.

3. Press the crown of the head forward, and with the toes tucked, press the heels back. Reach the heart forward and slide the shoulders towards the waist. Have the chin and neck in a neutral position, and look down 1-2 feet in front of the hands.

4. Breathe and hold for 1-4 breaths.

5. To release, bend the knees to the floor into child pose.

Benefits: Plank pose builds upper and core body strength, lengthens and strengthens the spine, and invigorates the body and mind.

Contraindications: Recent or chronic injury to the arms, back or shoulders.

Modifications: A) Bend both knees to the floor. B) Have the forearms flat to the floor with the fingers pointing forward.

Warrior III or Virabhadrasana III

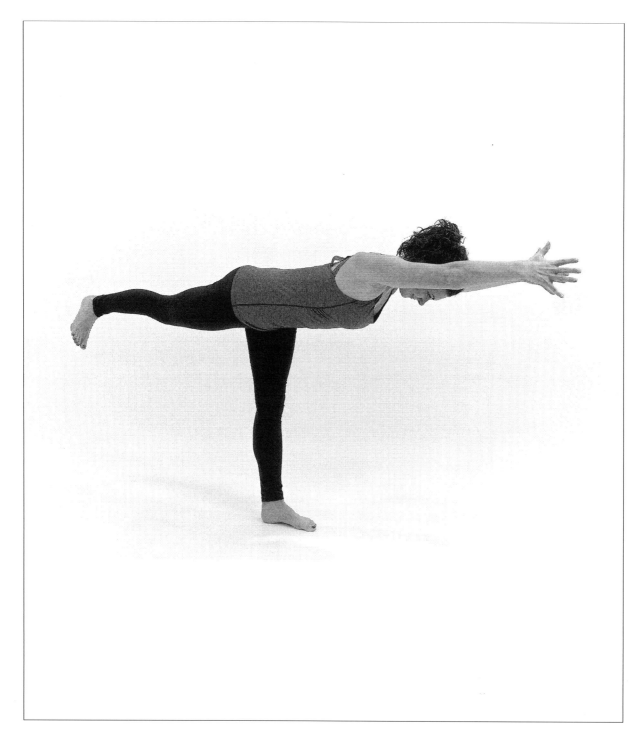

Invoke the intense gaze of a warrior launching into battle in this challenging balancing pose. Reach out and engage your core strength to let yourself fly high in warrior III.

Instructions

1. From mountain pose, step the right foot 1-2 feet forward and shift all of your weight onto this leg. Look down at the floor about 5 feet in front of you, and stare at a point for balance.

2. Inhale the arms over your head in an "H" position.

3. As you exhale, lift the left leg up and back, hinging at the hips to lower the arms and torso down towards the floor. Strongly engage the standing right leg, pressing the foot into the floor, and pulling up on the kneecap.

4. Reach out through the left toes, fingers and the crown, making one straight line. Work on sliding the shoulders in towards the waist and reaching the heart forward.

5. Breathe and hold for 2-6 breaths.

6. To release, inhale the arms up to lower the leg back to the floor and step both feet together back into mountain pose.

7. Repeat on the other side.

Benefits: Warrior III improves balance, memory, and concentration and tones and invigorates the whole body.

Contraindications: Recent or chronic injury to the legs, hips, back or shoulders.

Variations: A) Hold on to opposite elbows with the arms over your head. B) Bring the arms out to the sides. C) Place your hands on your hips, D) Interlace the fingers, pointing the index finger up.

Tree or Vrikshasana

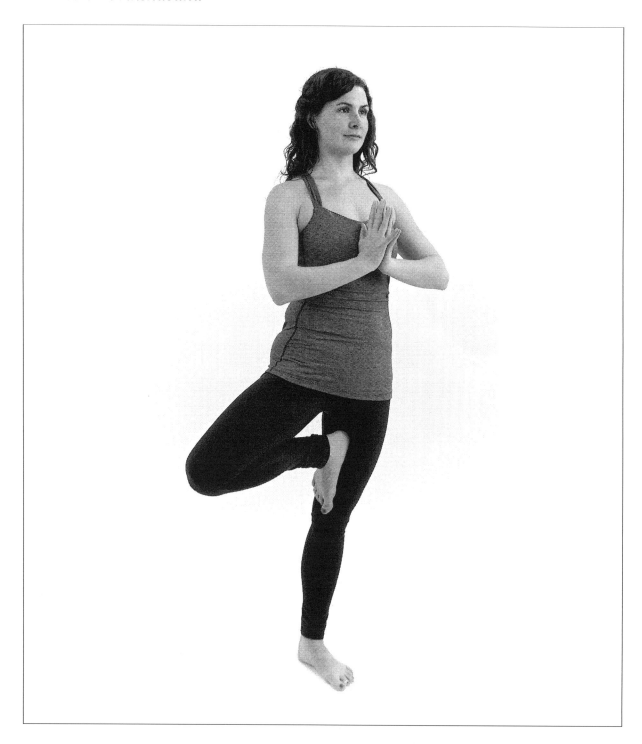

Send your roots deep down into the standing leg of tree pose to remain stable and focused even as you bend in the winds of change and inner struggle.

Instructions

1. From mountain pose, bend the right knee, shifting all the weight into the left leg. Turn the right knee to the right wall, resting the heel against the left leg.

2. Look down at the floor, and stare at one point. Slowly slide the right foot up the left leg as high up as you can maintain your balance. When you are balanced here, slowly bring the palms together in prayer position in front of the heart. If you need more stability, reach the arms out wide to the sides.

3. Keep staring at your focal point on the floor. Strongly engage the standing left leg, pressing the foot into the floor, pulling up on the kneecap and hugging the leg in towards your midline. Keep the right knee bent 90 degrees towards the side wall. The shoulders are down and back, the chest is pressing forward, and the crown of the head is lifted high.

4. If you are very balanced here, try the next stage by inhaling the arms over the head. The arms can be in an "H" position, the fingers can be interlaced with the index finger pointed up, or you can have the palms together with the thumbs crossed. The fingers are reaching up, and the shoulders are down and back.

5. Breathe and hold for 4-6 breaths.

6. To release, slowly exhale the arms down, and then release the legs back into mountain.

7. Repeat on the other side.

Benefits: Tree pose increases balance, focus, memory, and concentration and strengthens the ankles and knees.

Contraindications: Recent or chronic knee or hip injury.

Modifications: Practice next to a wall, placing a hand on the wall for support.

Upward Boat or Paripurna Navasana

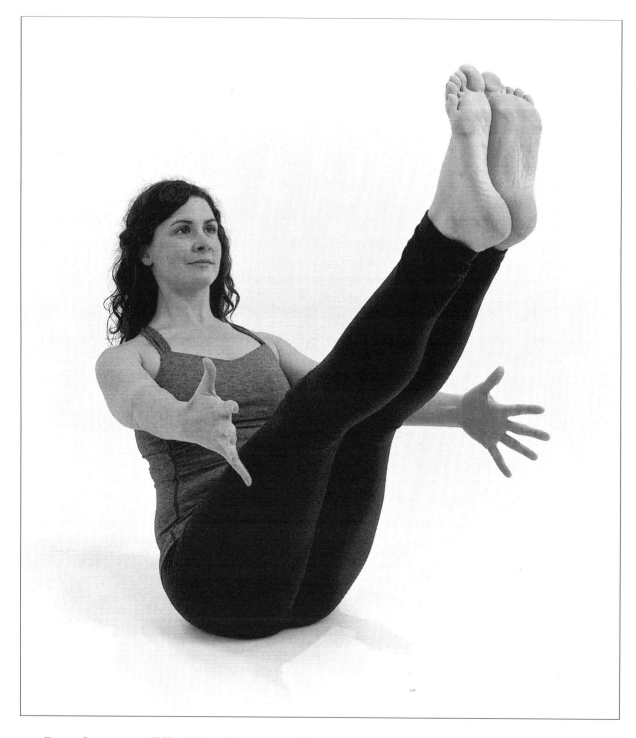

Stare down your difficulties with a strong, focused gaze in this core-strengthening pose. Cultivate a bold and strong inner will in upward boat, connect with the core of your being, and radiate your strength outwards.

Instructions

1. From a seated position, bend the knees, bringing the feet flat to the floor with the legs together. Slide the hands behind your hips with the fingers pointed forward and elbows bent away from you.

2. Reach the elbows back as you reach the sternum forward. Lean back to lift the heels an inch or two off the floor. Ground down through the sitting bones, and lengthen up through the crown of the head.

3. Slowly begin to straighten the legs, kicking out through the heels, lifting the legs up as high as comfortable. Release the arms forward, parallel to the floor with the palms facing each other. Keep the heart lifted and let the shoulders release down and back. Gaze at your toes.

4. Breathe and hold for 2-6 breaths. Put as much effort into lifting the chest as you are in lifting the legs.

5. To release, exhale and bend the knees, lowering the feet back to the floor.

Benefits: Boat pose tones and strengthens the abdominal muscles, improves balance and confidence, and stretches the backs of the legs.

Contraindications: Recent or chronic injury to the abdomen, knees, hips, arms or shoulders.

Modifications: A) To make the pose easier, keep the hands on the floor or interlace the hands behind the knees. B) Wrap a yoga strap around the feet and hold onto the strap with both hands.

Variations: Interlace the middle and index fingers around the big toes.

Using Dynamic Movements

DHYANA - ABSORBED STATE OF MIND

As your ability to focus and concentrate (dharana) increases, you will naturally progress towards dhyana, a state of meditation or deep mental absorption. (It is easy to get these two terms confused as to their similar Sanskrit spelling.) Concentration evolves into meditation simply by sustaining the focus of the mind for an unbroken amount of time. If you can keep your focus for over a minute, you are moving into the absorbed state of dhyana.

Know that both dharana and dhyana are higher stages of yogic practice, and while they sound simple, they are not easy to practice. As you learned in the last lesson, dharana requires a great deal of focus and willpower, and because dhyana is a higher stage of practice, it requires even more focus and willpower. Practicing dhyana will make you acutely aware of the constant clutter of thoughts arising in your mind, which makes this yogic practice an exceptional tool for examining your inner world and attaining a mastery over your mental thoughts.

The benefits of an absorbed state of mind are vast. Meditation has been shown to reduce stress, improve quality of life, and to increase one's overall sense of well-being. Studies have shown meditation to be effective in reducing blood pressure, lowering breath rate, and helping with depression, anxiety, panic attacks, and insomnia. Recent research has shown through MRI scans that meditation affects the brain on a physical level, increasing the overall size of the brain and strengthening the areas of the brain that are activated during states of focused absorption.

VINYASA

The synchronizing of physical movement with your breath in yoga is called vinyasa. This technique allows you to create a deeper absorption of awareness and to create a moving meditation.

Vinyasa also supports moving into and out of the asanas through the muscular breathing mechanisms. An inhalation naturally expands the belly and ribs and, with proper alignment, will lengthen the spine and encourage expansion. An exhalation naturally contracts the abdomen and torso and encourages retraction. In general, inhale when you move into a pose, move against gravity, create upward movements, or arch the spine. Exhale as you move out of a posture, move with gravity, create downward movements, or round the spine.

Vinyasa is best used in warmups and the sun salutation series. Some styles of yoga use vinyasa through the entire practice, which can often sacrifice proper alignment for moving quickly through the poses. However, the repetition of poses and movement with the breath does build familiarity, create mastery, build strength, and increase body heat.

At first, the synchronizing of movement with your breath in vinyasa can be a bit discombobulating. Once you get the hang of it and can establish a rhythm that works for your body, vinyasa will ultimately deepen your focus and awareness.

Do not sacrifice proper alignment to quickly move through a sequence. Slow down and take extra breaths if necessary. Vinyasa movement is best supported with the Ujjayi Pranayama breathing that we will learn next.

UJJAYI PRANAYAMA

Ujjayi Pranayama is called the victory or ocean-sounding breath because you make an ocean sound in your throat by contracting the glottis with the inhalation and exhalation. Ujjayi Pranayama aids in concentration and is very balancing and grounding during asana. This is a great pranayama to use to tune out any auditory distractions in your environment. Ujjayi Pranayama is also a healing breath that increases oxygen levels, strengthens the lungs, helps to purify the body of toxins, and increases the flow of prana energy through the body.

PRACTICE SESSION
Ujjayi Pranayama: The Ocean-Sounding Breath

To practice, come into easy pose or sukhasana (learned in Lesson 1). This pranayama is done through the nose, but it is helpful to begin practicing breathing through the mouth. To make the ocean sound, whisper the syllable "h," feeling the contraction in your throat. Keep this contraction engaged on the inhalation and exhalation. After a couple of breaths, try to close the mouth, breathing through the nose while still making the ocean sound in your throat.

Try to make the ocean sound as loud as possible without straining the throat. Focus your attention on the sound, letting it calm and soothe your mind. Practice this breathing technique for 3-5 minutes at the start of this lesson's practice.

Yoga meditation

To practice a basic yoga-based meditation, sit in a comfortable position, either cross-legged on the floor or in a chair. Sit up tall with the spine straight, the shoulders relaxed and the chest open. Rest the hands on the knees with the palms facing up. Lightly touch the index finger to the thumb. Relax the face, jaw, and belly. Let the tongue rest on the roof of the mouth, just behind the front teeth. Allow the eyes to lightly close.

Breathe slowly, smoothly and deeply in and out through the nose. Let the inhale start in the belly and then rise gently up into the chest. As the breath slows and deepens, let go of any thoughts or distractions, and allow the mind to focus on the breath. Feel the breath as it moves in and out of the body, through the nose, throat, windpipe and lungs. Feel the body as it rises and falls with each breath. Bring as much of your awareness and attention to your body and breath as possible with each moment. As the thoughts return to the mind, let them go, and return the focus to the body and breath.

Practice this meditation for 10-20 minutes before or after practicing ujjayi pranayama at the start of this lesson's practice.

Surya Namaskar: The Sun Salutation

Often considered the core of hatha yoga practice, Sun Salutations are traditionally practiced at sunrise to warm and energize the body. The classical series is used in most hatha yoga traditions with the exception of Ashtanga or power yoga. Sun salutations are practiced 2-6 times in a row and are traditionally practiced at sunrise. I recommend you start slow and focus on the alignment of each pose in the vinyasa, and then slowly move faster through the sequence until you can do one breath with each pose.

Contraindication: Recent or chronic injury to the back, knees, hips or unmedicated high blood pressure.

You can practice this session by itself or incorporate it with any previous practice sessions or previously learned poses. Please start your practice with the warm-up sequence we learned in Lesson 1, and practice Ujjayi Pranayama as much as possible through the entire practice.

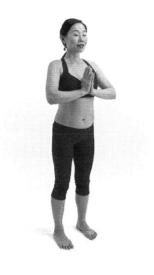

1. Start in Mountain with the palms together.

A. Place the feet together or 3-4 inches apart, parallel, and facing forward.

B. The palms are lightly pressed together with the shoulders back and down, and the chest presses in towards the thumbs.

C. The crown of the head lifts up, and the chin is parallel to the floor.

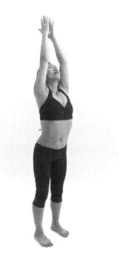

2. Inhale and sweep the arms up with palms together.

A. Stay in Mountain alignment.

B. Look up at the thumbs.

C. Lift out of the waist, reaching up towards the sky.

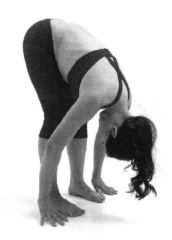

3. Exhale into Forward Fold.

A. Press the palms to the floor; if necessary, bend the knees slightly. If you have the flexibility, bring the fingertips in line with the toes.

B. Reach the forehead in towards the legs.

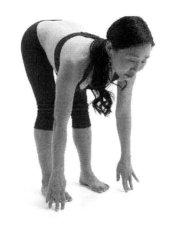

4. Inhale and lift into Half Forward Fold.

A. Lift the torso high enough to create a slight arch in the spine. Slide the hands up the legs for support if necessary.

B. Bring the eyes to the forehead. Reach the tailbone back and the head towards the wall in front.

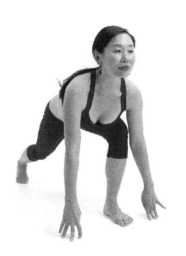

5. Exhale and step the right foot back into High Lunge.

A. Make sure the left knee is directly over the ankle and the toes and knees are pointing forward.

B. Shoulders are back and down, the chest presses forward, crown lifts up, and the back leg is straight.

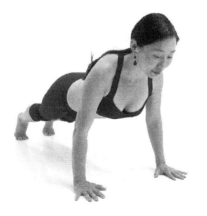

6. Inhale and step the left foot back into Plank.

A. The body is one straight line and in a push-up position.

B. Press the heels and tailbone back, and reach the crown of the head forward.

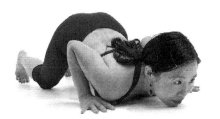

7. Exhale slowly down into Caterpillar.

A. Bend the knees to the floor, and bend the elbows to lower the chin and chest to the floor.

B. Reach the hips up towards the sky, arching the back.

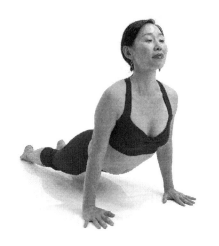

8. Inhale into Upward Facing Dog.

A. Scoop the chest forward, straighten the arms, and roll onto the tops of the feet.

B. Reach the crown of the head up, press the chest forward, and lift the hips and legs off of the floor. Bend the elbows slightly if it feels like you are straining the low back.

9. Exhale into Downward Facing Dog.

A. Tuck the toes under and lift the hips up and back.

B. Press firmly into the hands and arms to press the hips back. Let the head hang from the neck. Press the heels into the floor. The legs are straight or can be slightly bent to flatten the back.

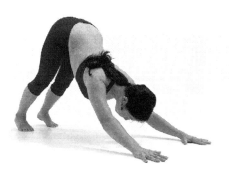

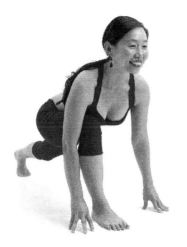

10. Inhale and step right forward into High Lunge.

A. Step the right foot forward between the two hands. Adjust the leg so that the knee is directly over the ankle and the toes and knee are pointing forward.

B. Keep the back leg straight as you sink the hips down. The crown lifts up, and the chest and gaze are forward.

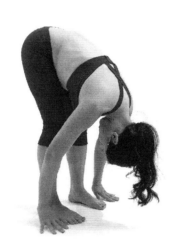

11. Exhale and step into Forward Fold.

A. Press the palms to the floor; if necessary bend the knees slightly. If you have the flexibility, bring the fingertips in line with the toes.

B. Reach the forehead in towards the legs.

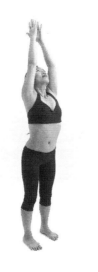

12. Inhale and sweep the arms up with palms together.

A. Have the legs and torso in Mountain alignment.

B. Look up at the thumbs.

C. Lift out of the waist, reaching up towards the sky.

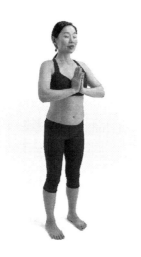

13. Exhale and bring the palms together in Mountain.

A. Pause here and take a few slow deep breaths to come back to your center.

B. Repeat the sun salutation sequence again or move on to practicing other poses.

Where To Go From Here

Yoga is a journey and a process; it is not a destination or a competition. There is no goal to achieve besides being completely present with where you are in your practice. Accept your body's limitations, and honor what it can and can't do, but don't let that be an excuse to minimize what you can achieve with yoga. With that in mind, you can go deeper into the journey of yoga through one or more of the following options.

Increase the intensity and challenge of the poses

There are three ways to increase the intensity of your practice: (1) hold postures for longer and longer periods of time; (2) slowly build your practice up to more advanced and challenging postures; (3) move more quickly between postures.

Use your breath as a way to time how long you are holding the poses, and slowly work on increasing the number of breaths in every pose or just a few favorite poses. When holding a pose, you want to be in a state of calm inner focus. When that calm inner focus is lost, it is time to come out of the pose.

Move slowly into any challenging postures while keeping the mind focused on the breath and the body. Feel what is happening in the body without the temptation to react, judge, or criticize. Take yourself right to your edge, breathe some more, and see if you can go just a tiny bit more. Give yourself permission to bail out at any time if the body (not the mind) is saying a big "no." Challenging postures can bring up strong emotions, and it is important to be in a safe environment so these emotions can be fully expressed and released from the body.

You can increase the speed of your movements to create heat, intensity and endurance, but do not move faster than one breath to one movement. Moving too quickly through vinyasa movements can compromise the alignment and structural integrity of the poses and potentially lead to injury.

Learn new yoga poses

You have learned a comprehensive list of yoga poses in this book, but there are many more poses and variations of poses that you can explore. The best way to approach a new yoga pose, especially a challenging one, is with a playful and open heart. You should practice new poses by themselves and then add them to your practice when you feel ready. See the bibliography for a list of resources to learn new yoga poses and practices.

Try a new sequence

There are some styles of yoga that have a set sequence from which you do not vary. Other styles of yoga never do the same sequence twice. I personally love to try out new combinations of yoga poses, as this changes how each pose feels and how I feel after the practice. You can modify any of the sequences in this book, create your own sequence from scratch, or find sequences in other books and on the internet (see the bibliography for references). Structure your yoga practice to start with simple and easy poses, and move toward more complex and challenging poses.

Practice yoga frequently

One of the best methods to deepen and strengthen your yoga practice is to practice yoga as frequently as possible. Having a daily practice is highly revered in yoga, but even a few times a week will be highly beneficial.

While most yoga classes are 60-90 minutes long, your daily practice can be shorter. Practicing just 10-15 minutes each day is better than practicing 90 minutes once a week. Practicing yoga frequently will accelerate your sense of familiarity and mastery of the poses. Practicing frequently will also be more effective in improving the flexibility and strength of the body.

Deepen your inner focus with pratyahara

Pratyahara translates directly as "sense withdrawal" and is the pivotal point in the practice of yoga where the path leads from the exterior to the interior landscape of the body. By withdrawing our attention from the external environment, and by focusing inwards on the breath and sensations, we still the mind and increase our awareness of the body. With this awareness and focus we can move deeper into the practice of yoga, learning to move through our limitations, fears and expectations. The key to practicing pratyahara is observing the body, breath and sensations as a detached witness, as if you were watching and feeling someone else's body. Used with compassion and discipline, pratyahara enriches the practice of yoga and leads to deeper stages of concentration and meditation.

Join a class/find an instructor

Once you are comfortable with many of the basic postures presented in this book, you may want to venture out into the community and attend a yoga class. Many studios offer a one time or first time fee that is affordable and/or free to new students, which gives you the opportunity to attend classes at more than one location and to try out different instructors to find the one that meets your own personal needs and goals. An instructor can provide assistance and guidance with asana, pranayama, and meditation.

A good teacher will also answer questions, make sure that you have proper alignment, and that you are getting the most benefit from your practice.

Explore and practice yoga philosophy

The main philosophy of yoga is simple: mind, body and spirit are all one and cannot be clearly separated. Yet, there is a multitude of philosophical ideas developed by looking into the deeper dimensions of the body, mind and spirit. We will briefly discuss a few of the main yogic philosophical ideas here.

The yamas and niyamas are moral, ethical and societal guidelines and internal practices for the practicing yogi. The yamas are all expressed in the positive, and thus become emphatic descriptions of how a yogi behaves and relates to her world when truly immersed in the unitive state of yoga. While we may not strive to reach such a pure state ourselves, the *yamas* are still highly relevant and valued guides to lead a conscious, honest and ethical life. The *niyamas* extend the ethical codes of conduct of the yamas to the practicing yogi's internal environment of body, mind and spirit. The practice of *niyama* helps us maintain a positive environment in which to grow, and it gives us the self-discipline and inner strength necessary to progress along the path of yoga. Below are the ten yamas and niyamas as described in Patanjali's *Yoga Sutras*:

• *Ahimsa* (non-harming) is the practice of non-violence, which includes physical, mental, and emotional violence towards others and the self.

• *Satya* (truthfulness) urges us to live and speak our truth at all times.

• *Asteya* (non-stealing) is best defined as not taking what is not freely given.

• *Brahmacharya* (continence) states that when we have control over our physical impulses of excess, we attain knowledge, vigor, and increased energy.

• *Aparigraha* (non-coveting) urges us to let go of everything that we do not need, possessing only what is necessary.

• *Shaucha* (purification) is a central aim of many yogic techniques to create a healthy body and a pure state of mind.

• *Samtosha* (contentment) is not craving for what we do not have as well as not coveting the possessions of others.

• *Tapas* (asceticism) is a yogic practice of intense self-discipline and attainment of willpower.

• *Svadhyaya* (self-study) is the ability to see our true divine nature through the contemplation of our life's lessons and through the meditation on the truths revealed by seers and sages.

• *Ishvara Pranidhana* (devotion) is the dedication, devotion, and surrender of the fruits of one's practice to a higher power.

The Bhagavad Gita, the most treasured and famous of India's spiritual texts, is a dialogue between Prince Arjuna and Sri Krishna, Arjuna's charioteer, friend, and council. The story opens to the scene of a battlefield just prior to the start of a colossal war, with Arjuna asking Krishna for guidance. The resulting conversation between Arjuna and Krishna develops into a discourse on the nature of the soul, the purpose of one's life, and many other fundamental philosophical tenets. Below are seven key philosophical concepts discussed between Krishna and Arjuna in this epic tale:

• *Jaya* (self-mastery) is the ability to harness and control your physical, mental, and spiritual well-being. The attainment of self-mastery can be used to produce right action (dharma) and desired personal changes at will. Self-mastery also creates a deep satisfaction with life and a strong sense of self-confidence.

• *Maya* (illusion) is the power that distorts our vision to see things other than the way they truly are. Maya is often so strong that we do not see or realize this distortion or clouding of our view. Unless we are enlightened, we can assume maya is always present, and we can always work on establishing a higher perspective with which to view the troubles of our lives. Our yoga practice can help pierce the veil of maya and understand the distortions of its lens through the conscious cultivation of clarity, wisdom, and open-mindedness.

• *Dharma* (right action or duty) is a combination of one's personal obligations, purpose in life, talents, and societal duties. Your dharma is highly influenced by your karma, your genetics, and the culture and worldview into which you are born. Following your dharma involves acknowledging your talents and using those skills to take the most effective path to reach the goal or purpose of your life.

• *Atman* (true self, soul) is the innermost soul or spirit that resides in everyone. The atman is described as being a small connected piece of the ultimate oneness of the universe.

• *Samsara* (continuous flow) is the endless cycle of birth, life, death, and reincarnation. The aim of enlightenment is to escape the cycle of samsara.

• *Vairagya* (dispassion) is freedom from craving all objects of desire, both material objects and spiritual experiences. The yogis' technique for reducing desire is to cultivate vairagya through the conscious severing of our attachments to the objects of this world. Vairagya applies both to our likes and dislikes, with the ideal goal of seeing both sweet and bitter fruits of life as the same. The practice of detachment needs to be balanced with willful effort (abhyasa) and must never be an excuse to abandon one's worldly duties and obligations.

• *Upekkha* (equanimity) is the power to maintain our center, peace, and equanimity in the face of adversity and challenge. It is the emotionally detached state of one who witnesses without becoming emotionally involved. It is a virtue and an attitude to be cultivated, as opposed to simple indifference or lack of interest. The more enlightened yogi is one who, with spiritual intelligence, acts equally towards well-wishers, enemies, the envious, friends, saintly persons as well as the sinful.

The law of karma is the universal spiritual concept of reaping what you sow. Karma is the future consequences of one's current intentions, thoughts, behaviors and actions. While the karma you currently create become the seeds of future life experiences, your karma is not your fate. You have the ability to consciously choose how you respond and react to karmically generated events, thus reducing the current impact of your karma and reducing or eliminating future karma. This is both a psychological and physical practice, with the mental attitude much more powerful than the physical deed.

The law of karma is connected to the constant, changing physical world the yogis call samsara, the spinning wheel of life and death. This wheel is said to have six spokes: virtue and vice, pleasure and pain, attachment and aversion. These spokes are the types of karma that bind us to the wheel and keep it spinning. The goal is to break these karmic spokes to become liberated from the mundane and suffering world of samsara.

Explore the subtle body

The ancient yogis discovered a rich inner world that is composed of life force energy or prana. This energy can be experienced, accessed, and manipulated in various ways. Once you are comfortable with the external engagement of the yoga poses, then you can bring your focus inwards to the subtle or energetic body.

Prana (life force energy) comes into the body from the food we eat, the air we breathe, and from absorbing the energies of the earth and heavens. This mystical energy flows through our bodies and generates our every action – from gross physical movements to minute biochemical processes. Prana travels through thousands of tiny channels called nadis to every cell in the body. The three main nadis in the body are the ida, pingala and sushumna, which all start at the base of the spine and travel upwards to the head. The ida and pingala nadis crisscross each other as they spiral upwards and connect to opposite nostrils, while the sushumna travels straight up the spine to the crown of the head.

The **chakras** are located where the ida and pingala nadis cross each other and intersect with the sushumna channel. The chakras connect with the thousands of minor nadis and are thus responsible for the distribution and circulation of prana throughout the whole body.

Hatha yoga was developed to circulate, cultivate, and control prana and to activate and channel kundalini (dormant spiritual energy) up the sushumna nadi to the crown chakra. Asana cultivates and circulates prana in the body and strengthens the nadis. Pranayama, the use of various breathing techniques, controls and cultivates the prana and purifies the nadis.

Koshas (sheaths) are five coverings that veil the light of our atman (highest self). The koshas are visualized like the layers of an onion and form a barrier from realizing our true nature of bliss and oneness with the universe. Yoga is the tool to peel back these layers to bring our awareness deeper and deeper into our bodies, eventually reaching the innermost core, our True Self. When we can clearly see through the layers of the koshas, we then attain a state of yoga, oneness with the universe.

There are three primary ***Bandhas*** (locks) used in hatha yoga to locally contain the prana in the torso and concentrate it in the three main nadis. The three bandhas (mula, uddiyana and jalandhara) are typically used in advanced pranayama, but these bandhas can also be effectively employed in asana practice.

Mudras (gesture, seal) are subtle physical movements of the hands, face, and/or body. Complex mudras involve the whole body in a combination of asana, pranayama, bandha and visualization, while simple mudras range from hand positions to meditation techniques. The purpose of a mudra is to activate and create a circuit of prana in the body. This circuit channels the prana in a specific way to create a subtle effect on koshas and to regulate and awaken the prana, chakras and kundalini. Mudras are used only after proficiency in asana, pranayama, and bandha has been achieved and when one has obtained some cultivation and awareness of prana.

Embrace yoga as a lifestyle

The potential for yoga to transform your life is infinite. Even without trying, practicing yoga on a consistent basis will slowly influence your life through the activities you pursue, the friends with whom you associate, and the foods that you eat. By consciously incorporating the philosophy of yoga into your lifestyle, you will further be able to change and overcome many obstacles that you face in your life. You may even learn to practice yoga "off the mat"– the skill of becoming calm, centered and present on your yoga mat will eventually seep into every other area of your life.

Afterword

I like to end my yoga classes by chanting "Om, shanti, shanti, shanti" and by giving my translation of this ancient mantra as "May peace reside within your heart, may this peace stay with you throughout the rest of your day, and may this peace spread from you, to others, to eventually the whole world."

If I was in your presence I would also add to the above: "Namaste. I bow to the place in you where the entire universe resides. I honor the place in you of love, of light, of truth, of peace. I bow to your divine spirit, to your inherent buddhahood, to the great ball of sunshine that radiates from your heart."

Thank you for taking this journey of yoga with me. I hope that this book has been helpful and that it will continue to encourage and support you on the path of yoga in the days ahead. If you have benefited from this book I would be honored if you left a review on this book's Amazon.com page.

Glossary

Ahimsa is a vow to practice nonviolence and harmlessness to yourself and others.

Aparigraha is a vow to practice non-coveting and greedlessness.

Asanas are the yoga postures, poses or positions.

Ashram is a dedicated retreat or secluded place where yoga and meditation are taught and practiced.

Asmita is the Sanskrit word for ego and individuality.

Asteya is a vow to practice non-stealing and not taking what is not freely given.

Atman is the true Self or inner spirit that is connected to everything in the universe.

Bhakti yoga is a major path of yoga that is focused on devotional practices.

Brahmacharya is often translated as celibacy, but can also mean purity, chastity, and non-lusting.

Brahman is the divine oneness of all things.

Buddhi is the intellect and thinking part of the mind.

Chakras are energy centers located along the spine that are described as "whirling disks of light." Each of the seven chakras are said to radiate a specific color and spiritual quality, and are associated with a corresponding psychological, physical, and emotional state.

Crown of the Head is the top of your head towards the back, directly above the center of the spine.

Dharana is mental focus and concentration used to hold the mind's awareness on one point.

Dharma is one's role and purpose in life.

Dhyana is meditation.

Guru is a spiritual teacher that one commits to studying under.

Hatha yoga is a major path of yoga that focuses on spiritual attunement through physical exercises and practices.

Ishvar-pranidhana is the dedication of your practice to something that is greater than yourself.

Jnana yoga is the yogic path of knowledge or wisdom.

Karma is the universal spiritual concept of reaping what you sow.

Karma yoga is the yogic path of living in the world without striving for any external rewards.

Kundalini is a stored spiritual energy in the body that is often compared to a snake lying coiled at the base of the spine, waiting to be awakened.

Mantra is a Sanskrit prayer that is repeated or chanted as a form of meditation.

Meditation is a technique of stilling and calming the mind by focusing all attention on one object.

Mudras are specific subtle muscular engagements of the hands, head or whole body to cultivate and increase energy in the body.

Namaste is a salutation that translates as "the divine in me honors the divine in you." The expression is often used at the end of a yoga class accompanied by the gesture of holding the palms together in front of the heart and gently bowing.

Niyamas are the internal practices or moral observances for the practicing yogi. The specific niyamas vary with each major path of yoga and usually total five in number.

Om or Aum is the vibration and sound of the universe in a state of oneness. Chanting this mantra connects one to this oneness.

Prana translates into "life force energy" and is the sense of energy that we experience in our body.

Pranayama is a breathing practice that is used to control, cultivate, and modify the prana in the body.

Pratyahara is a state of inner focus achieved through removing our attention of our sense organs.

Raja yoga is a major path of yoga that focuses on meditation and mental control.

Santosha is a vow to practice contentment.

Satya is a vow to practice truthfulness and honesty.

Samadhi is a state of enlightenment.

Shauca is a vow to practice purity, and both inner and outer cleanliness.

Sitting Bones are the two ischial tuberosities or bony protrusions at the bottom of the two hip bones that form the pelvis. In a seated position these are the bones that press against the floor.

Svadhyaya is a commitment to study oneself as well as to study the ancient scriptures and teachings of yoga.

Swami is a title of respect for an accomplished and dedicated yoga teacher.

Tantra yoga is a path of yoga that uses ritual, visualization, chanting, asana, and strong breathing practices to tap highly charged kundalini energy in the body.

Tapas is a yogic practice of intense self-discipline and attainment of willpower.

Vinyasa is a flow of yoga postures that are synced with breath to create a continuous movement.

Yamas are the moral, ethical and societal guidelines for the practicing yogi. The specific yamas vary with each major path of yoga and usually total five in number.

Yoga is any practice that brings the practitioner into a state of oneness of body, mind and spirit.

Yogi is someone who practices yoga. A female practitioner is sometimes called a yogini.

Resources

WEBSITES

• YogaBasics.com can be an essential part of developing your own yoga practice and will assist you in further developing your knowledge and practice of yoga. From the beginner to the intermediate and advanced student, YogaBasics.com provides you with the essentials you need to move beyond your current abilities.

• YouTube.com has over a half million videos on yoga. Most of these are short and are not professionally filmed, but they are all free to stream. You can also find videos for very specific issues and videos that focus on individual poses.

• YogaJournal.com features interesting articles from its past magazine issues and has professionally filmed videos, but most of the site's content is not very friendly or useful for beginner students.

BOOKS

• Hatha Yoga Illustrated by Brooke Boon is a good yoga pose encyclopedia of 77 postures with full color photos and clear step-by-step instructions.

• Yogaflows by Mohini Chatlani is a wonderful book full of creative yoga pose sequences.

• Yoga Anatomy by Leslie Kaminoff is a great book if you are interested in a deeper understanding of the anatomical foundations of the yoga poses.

• Yoga as Medicine by Timothy McCall is a helpful guide to using yoga as a therapeutic tool for healing common diseases and complaints.

• Yoga Body by Mark Singleton is a fascinating history of modern yoga.

• Bhagavad Gita is the one of the primary yogic scriptures, and the wonderful translation by Eknath Easwaran has a great philosophic overview for each chapter.

VIDEOS

The video DVDs listed below are all suitable for beginning level students. Each DVD has a slightly different focus, approach and types of yoga poses.

• Basic Yoga Workout for Dummies

• A.M./P.M. Yoga for beginners

• Yoga For Beginners

About the Author

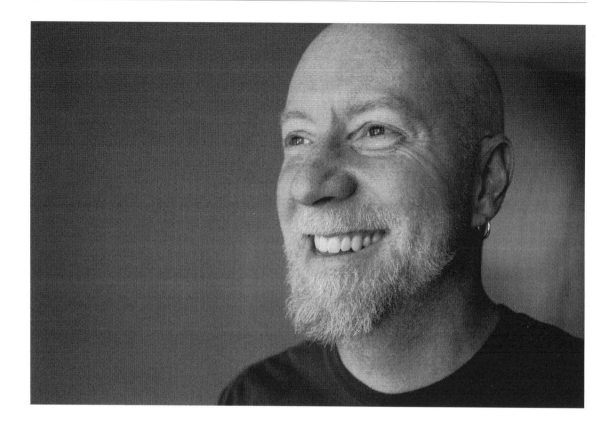

If Timothy Burgin's teaching philosophy could be summed up in one sentence, it would be Rusty Wells' quote: "Who cares if you can touch your toes if you can't touch your heart?" When Timothy started practicing yoga 22 years ago, he couldn't even touch his toes, but yoga certainly touched his heart. Timothy's love for yoga has since led him to complete over 500 hours of yoga teacher training, create multiple yoga based businesses, and instruct thousands of yoga students all over the world.

Timothy's greatest love is sharing the teachings and practices of yoga with others. Trained and certified in the Kripalu and Prankriya yogic traditions, Timothy has both the knowledge and experience to guide his students deep into the experience of yoga and to address their individual needs through gentle assists, variations, and pose modifications. He possesses a unique and wonderful combination of centeredness, authenticity, thoughtfulness and playfulness. Timothy's students often describe him as a kind, compassionate, gentle and accessible yoga teacher.

Timothy deepened his knowledge and understanding of the physical body and its energetic and physiological systems when he completed his master's degree in acupuncture from the Santa Barbara College of Oriental Medicine. He brings his experience of healing and alternative medicine to his therapeutic yoga teachings.

Timothy's desire and mission to inspire and help people change their own lives led him to create Yogabasics.com, a place for the next generation of yoga practitioners to begin their journey. He hasn't forgotten how scary and intimidating it can be to start something new and to be vulnerable while learning. As a young college student in California, Timothy was called to the path of yoga after he reluctantly signed up for a class at the local university. "The Qi Gong class's prerequisite was yoga," he says with a sly grin, quickly adding, "I now see there were other plans for me." While fearful that a yoga class would be too challenging for his very inflexible 19-year old body, Timothy made it through his first class and subsequently fell in love with the practice.

Finding his home in Asheville, NC, Timothy continues to teach yoga classes and lead workshops and retreats internationally. Ever evolving, Timothy helps to keep the global yoga community breathing and moving through Yogabasics.com, with the intention of providing a comprehensive resource and guide for yoga, his yoga students, and the world.

In addition, Timothy is the founder of JapaMalaBeads.com, a company dedicated to producing and importing quality mala beads for prayer and meditation. Sensing the need from his students and the community for more intensive yoga practice time in exotic locations, Timothy formed Yoga Basics Retreats, the latest addition to the Yogabasics family. Timothy also the author of _Yoga For Beginners: A Quick-Start Guide to Practicing Yoga for New Students_.

35701541R00079

Made in the USA
Lexington, KY
20 September 2014